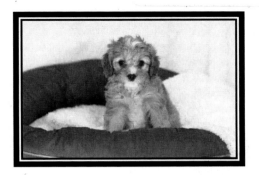

The Complete HAPPY Cavapoo Guide

Raise a Happy, Well-Mannered Dog and Avoid Dog Behavior Professionals for Life

- Dog Happiness Tips
- Techniques for a Well-behaved Cavapoo
- Prevent Behavior Issues
- Fulfill Your Puppy's Needs
- Be the Ideal Guardian
- Avoid Common Mistakes

Asia Moore

Dog Behavior Expert & Acclaimed Author

Copyrighted © 2020

Author: Asia Moore
www.K-9SuperHeroesDogWhispering.com
www.KnowsToNose.com
www.MustHavePublishing.com

Editor & Researcher: Alex Warrington, Ph.D.

Published by:
Worldwide Information Publishing
London
Great Britain
2020

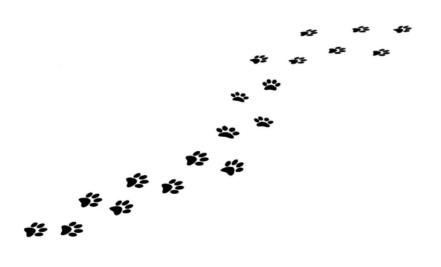

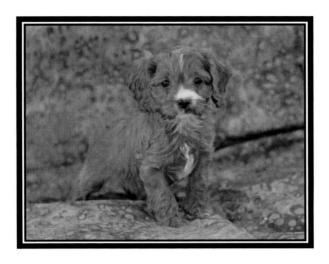

"Dogs are small rays of light caught on the Earth a short time to brighten our days."
— Unknown

Preface

It takes time, commitment, tenacity, consistency and knowledge to raise a happy and healthy Cavapoo that doesn't suffer from health and behavioral issues.

This book is NOT like most other breed-specific books, because we believe that it's far better for all parties concerned (human and canine) to **prevent** problems rather than suffering the frustrations of living with or learning how to eliminate problems and rehabilitate a Cavapoo that has already developed health or behavioral issues.

It is always better to prevent unwanted behaviors than to hope you, or someone else, may have what it takes to eliminate them in the future, after your family is at their wits end, your neighbors hate you, your friends no longer visit, your dog has been deemed dangerous, and you're having guilty thoughts of re-homing every time you drive past your local SPCA.

If you want a happy, well-mannered Cavapoo canine companion to be a loyal, valued member of your family, it absolutely matters how you raise your dog.

Every breed has uniquely different needs. Even those that were once working breeds that are now companion breeds.

For instance, a Border Collie is a very smart, high-energy dog that excels at the job of sheep herding. Therefore, if you expect this dog to sit around doing nothing all day while you're at work, you will most likely return to holes in your drywall, torn apart couches and a home that looks like it's been through a cyclone.

On the other hand, the Shih Tzu lap dog, which was originally only permitted to be owned by royalty, sat on silk pillows, was used to warm beds, has vastly different daily exercise requirements, and would be a poor choice for someone requiring a companion that could protect them from being mugged on streets ravaged by gang warfare.

The Cavapoo is a designer hybrid canine companion that is half Cavalier King Charles Spaniel and half Miniature Poodle. This means that learning the basics about both of these breeds will help you to determine if this is the right dog for you and your family.

Every dog breed has different talents and needs and when you decide to share your life with a particular breed, if you want a happy and well-adjusted companion, you must also be prepared to provide your dog with what he or she needs to be a happy member of your family.

Almost all canine problems, both mentally and physically, are a direct result of ignorance or unwillingness on the part of the human guardian to choose the right dog for their particular energy and lifestyle. It takes research, time and commitment to learn what each dog truly needs.

This book is uniquely different, and humans reading it need to clearly understand that the pages of this book are not all about describing what to do to eliminate problematic canine behaviors that have already occurred.

Rather, the main focus of this breed-specific book is to describe what the human guardian needs to understand and commit to doing on a daily basis in order to match the Cavapoo's needs, so that they can raise a happy, healthy and well-behaved dog that never has to experience behavioral issues.

Do not expect this book to be like all the others that set out endless correlations between specific mal-behaviors and what steps or actions the human guardian can take in an attempt to correct them.

In other words, this book is a totally new slant on raising a happy and healthy Cavapoo, because the main focus here is on the prevention of behavioral issues rather than addressing them after they have already surfaced.

About the Author

Asia Moore

Dog Behavior Expert & Acclaimed Author

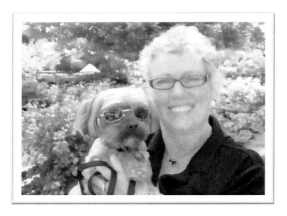

Ever since my first birthday, I was immersed in nature, and have always enjoyed a special connection with all creatures, both great and small. I learned to communicate and "talk" with many animals in their language, both wild and domesticated. At approximately the age of twelve, dogs began to become the main focus of my life, when I set about training and grooming my first puppy.

When friends and neighbors began to recognize how well behaved my dog was, and were subsequently impressed with all the tricks and routines she could perform, often without a spoken word, they asked me to train their dogs, too.

I've been so fortunate to have experienced the unconditional love of so many dogs over the years, all of who taught me many different life lessons. I began this journey with my first mixed breed ("Cindy") who protected me from my marauding brothers, then my mixed breed ("Pepper") who had an amazing human vocabulary and always knew when someone was not to be trusted, my Blue Heeler ("Bugsy") who would hike endless trails and swim miles with me, to my current loving Shih Tzu ("Boris") and all my clients' dogs in between.

Now, some 40 years later, and endless different breeds, including these patient and affectionate clowns of the dog world, and many hybrids and mutts, from tiny Chihuahuas to bouncing Belgians, a cascade of fur friends have passed through my life.

For the last 40 years, I have been managing my dog whispering, dog sitting and grooming businesses and have enjoyed countless experiences of working with dogs of all breeds and their guardians. It hasn't always been easy, and while I've had my fair share of struggles and setbacks, I've always loved and been passionate about what I do.

All these years of experience taught me invaluable lessons in all aspects of the human-canine relationship interaction. For instance, I learned how to effectively communicate with our canine friends, understand their needs and help them and their guardians lead a fulfilling and happy life together. *What could be better than that?*

Clients' dogs now remain the focal point of my dog whispering, sitting and grooming life, while I also focus on writing children's books and breed-specific books. I have so far authored over 300 books, where my goal is to pass on my knowledge and experience to all responsible dog owners (**Must Have Publishing.com**). At the same time, I continue to train human guardians, so that they can improve their relationships with their dogs and understand how to prevent and alleviate behavioral issues (**K-9 Super Heroes Dog Whispering.com**).

As well, I have recently added an additional online branch to my business, which I call "Knows To Nose" to help humans "know" how to choose the right dog "nose" for their energy and lifestyle, before they make the wrong decision and end up with troubling problems.

I am also often called upon to speak to groups about the changing roles for the canine population and how they now fit into our modern world. As well, I help humans and their chosen canines establish harmonious relationships with neighbors for those residing in multi-family living situations, such as apartment and condominium complexes.

I feel blessed that the canine world has been a major part of my life for so many years, as it never gets old. I continuously stay in touch with my clients through my business websites and personal consultations and I love how there is always room to learn more, because every unique dog brings new lessons to light and enhances everyone's life in untold, indescribable ways.

I'd like to thank you for purchasing "The Complete Happy Cavapoo Guide" and reassure you that the pages of this book contain the distilled knowledge of over 40 years experience, which, by the way, includes helping a Cavapoo suffering from anxiety about crossing over unfamiliar, slippery floor tiles.

When taken to heart, the knowledge, tips and techniques in this book can help you along your special journey inside the amazing world of our canine friends, so that you can know the unconditional love, special bond and joy that only our four-legged companions selflessly offer to us flawed humans.

Visit Asia online at the following locations:

www.K-9SuperHeroesDogWhispering.com
www.KnowsToNose.com
www.MustHavePublishing.com

Table of Contents

Chapter 1: Introduction

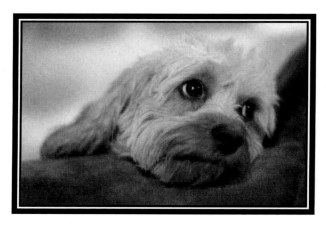

*"Properly trained, a man
can be dog's best friend."*
— Corey Ford

The purpose of this book is to focus on the important steps the humans in this relationship really need to be aware of and commit to providing in order to ensure that their Cavapoo companion can live a happy and healthy life, which in turn will ensure a happy relationship for everyone.

Even though humans and dogs have been relying on one another for more than 30,000 years, it's still highly important that you take an honest look at your life, and choose the companion that is best suited to your particular lifestyle.

Within the pages of this book you will find information to help you choose wisely by providing you with a clear understanding concerning whether or not YOU have what it takes to be the right match for raising a happy and well-mannered Cavapoo companion.

In addition, this book describes in detail what the human guardian needs to keep in mind and commit to doing on a daily basis in order to match this charming companion's needs, so that they can raise a happy, healthy and well-behaved dog that never has to experience behavioral issues.

All the information, suggestions, tips and advice given in this publication is the result of more than 40 years experience helping humans positively and effectively interact with the canine world.

If you take all that is written on these pages to heart, and regularly and consistently apply them, your sweet Cavapoo will be a happy family member that will not have to suffer from any behavioral problems. In other words, the focus is placed on prevention, rather than trying to correct any issues after they have surfaced.

Every Chapter of this book contains valuable information that will provide you with a solid understanding of the breed and the steps you need to take to raise a happy and well-behaved Cavapoo.

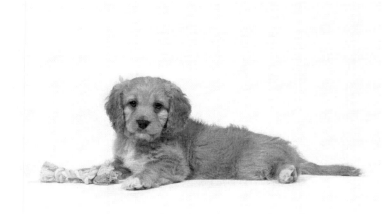

For instance, **Chapter 2** – *"Asia's Happiness Tips"* sets out a summary of what she personally believes makes for a happy Cavapoo and encourages you to ask yourself what YOU think would make this dog happy.

Chapter 3 – *"Overview of the Happy Cavapoo"* will outline vital statistics, coat colors and common features, intelligence, temperament and interesting secrets and facts that may not be commonly known. In order to raise a contented dog, you need to have some basic knowledge of the history of the Cavapoo breed, to help you choose wisely so that you are able to comprehend this dog's needs.

Chapter 4 – *"Healthy Cavapoo = Happy Dog"* is where you will find out what you need to know about medical care, safety and health issues that may affect this toy-sized breed, including common diseases and viruses, allergies and canine CPR procedures that could save a life. Needless to say, if your Cavapoo is not physically healthy, he or she will not be a happy canine companion for very long, because suffering from health-related issues will undoubtedly create a miserable and ill-mannered dog.

In **Chapter 5** – *"Let Your Dog BE a Happy Dog"*, you will find information about how to let your Cavapoo actually BE a dog, rather than attempting to turn them into a fur human, which can make for a very confused, unhappy and ill-mannered canine.

Chapter 6 – *"Every Happy Cavapoo Wants Exercise"*, first outlines some of the original history of this purebred dog that has become a companion; if you know what they were bred to do, you will better understand how important it is to commit to the daily exercise routines recommended in this book, without which the Cavapoo will not be happy for very long.

Chapter 7 – *"Feeding the Happy Cavapoo"*, is where you will find information about the structure of the canine jaw, various food options and feeding suggestions as well as treats to avoid for raising a happy and healthy companion.

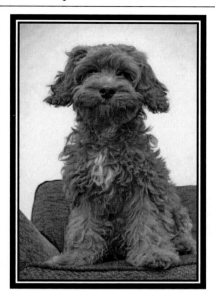

In **Chapter 8** – *"Care of the Happy Cavapoo"*, you will find travel safety tips, licensing, insurance, essential grooming procedures and important care of nails, ears, teeth and paws, all of which will help you to raise a happy Cavapoo. While this information might seem generic, imagine how you might feel going for months without washing your hair, cutting your nails or brushing your teeth. Unfortunately, that is the reality for many dogs, because their owners have not been properly advised with respect to the importance of good grooming habits. How happy and well behaved do you think such a poorly cared for Cavapoo would be? Be aware that the friendly, little Cavapoo with the ever-growing soft and silky or curly coat is high maintenance in the grooming department.

Chapter 9 – *"Are YOU the Ideal Happy Cavapoo Guardian?"* is concerned with asking yourself some serious questions, including whether your energy, activity, commitment and lifestyle matches what this hybrid needs to be happy and well behaved. It's vital for you to give serious consideration to these questions when considering this breed, because should you choose the wrong dog to share your life with, everybody will be miserable.

Chapter 10 – *"Humans Make a LOT of Stupid Mistakes"* outlines that far too often we humans, without even realizing it, are the cause of creating behavioral problems in our canine companions. You will find out what are some of the common mistakes to avoid (and the right thing to do!) when it comes to socialization, accidental rewards, fear of noises, the right collars, basic rules and boundaries, adolescent craziness and more. Simply being aware of the many mistakes we humans can often inadvertently be guilty of when raising our canine companions, can mean the difference between a Happy Cavapoo with no behavioral issues or a life of frustration and correction.

Chapter 11 – *"Happy Cavapoo Body Language"*, outlines the basics of learning canine body language, and will help you be safe around other dogs. Learning to properly "read" a dog's intentions can prevent an unwanted encounter with another canine or human, and this will help to ensure that everyone remains happy.

In Chapter 12 – *"Training Basics for a Happy Cavapoo"*, you will learn valuable training tips and routines that will help to keep your dog truly happy and well behaved for their entire life. It's no surprise that a properly trained companion will be a much happier companion that everyone enjoys being around, and will be far less likely to develop behaviour issues later in life. Developing a basic training program and learning to teach your dog commands and discipline is all part of starting your dog off on the right paw.

Chapter 13 – *"What If You Slip Up?"* is only necessary because we humans tend to get too busy and overwhelmed with the rigors of daily living, which means we sometimes forget to be consistent with providing what our particular dog may need to be happy. If you slip up, this Chapter has outlined a few of the more common behavioral issues and how to quickly get yourself back on track.

Chapter 14 – *"Surprise Bonus Chapter"* is a Question and Answer section containing a few human/canine situations, with humans asking questions and wise words from the perspective of the dog, which answers the questions. You will also find an amusing and educational true story about a happy dog that just refused to set one paw on the newly installed tiles in his family home.

Take heed humans, because when you honestly assess your own compatibility, lifestyle and energy level for being the right guardian for the Cavapoo, and are vigilant about following the advice and tips outlined in the following pages, you can raise a healthy and happy dog that will be a joy to live with and will never have to suffer from any behavioral issues.

Chapter 2: Asia's Happiness Tips

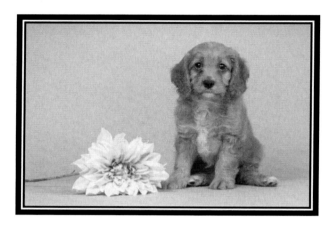

*"Dogs do speak, but only to
those who know how to listen."*
— Orhan Pamuk

The following few paragraphs are a summary of my own personal ramblings, beliefs, and ideas about what I think makes for a happy Cavapoo.

While I hope you may wholeheartedly agree, it's absolutely okay if you have other ideas, or if you may have an entirely different take on this subject, because we will all have our own "personal" ideas about what constitutes happiness for a sweet and playful Cavapoo, and if your ideas are different from mine, this does not mean that they are any less valid.

If you're considering sharing your life with the small, sturdy and fun-loving Cavapoo, and have never before really sat down and consciously thought about what would make this particular breed truly happy, while you may gain a little insight from reading about my own personal beliefs, I encourage you to take the time to do this exercise yourself. If you have a family, get them involved in this fun exercise, too.

When you take the time to sit with a piece of paper and pen and begin to write down what YOU think makes a Cavapoo happy, you may be surprised about what surfaces, and this simple exercise may inspire you and your family to discover new ways to bond with your dog, which will be the basis of having a truly happy relationship.

I'll help to get you started with the following question:
"What do you think would make a Cavapoo happy?"

I've shared the last 14 years of my life with a wonderfully loving and well behaved Shih Tzu and I believe that the very best start you can make, with respect to "happiness" when first bringing home your new Cavapoo puppy is to do all you can to reassure him or her that they are not alone (see below).

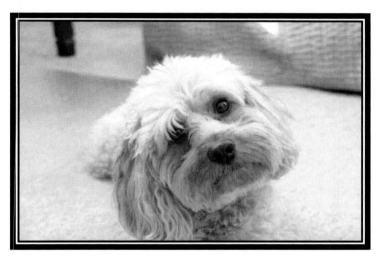

Happy New Surroundings

The puppy will be understandably nervous about the new and unfamiliar faces, surroundings and smells, and will be missing their mother, other siblings and everything in their environment they had grown used to during their first 8 to 10 weeks of life.

Make sure that you don't overwhelm your new puppy with too much all at once. For instance, close off rooms that you don't need access to and encourage your puppy to come to you as you wander about in a smaller space.

Happy Sleep Patterns

When it's time to go to bed, take your puppy outside for a bathroom break, and then make sure that you have a nice, cozy kennel all ready for your new puppy with a soft lining or blanket and place their new bedroom inside your room, so that they will be able to hear and see you.

Unless you want your Cavapoo to sleep on your bed when they're fully grown, even when they may have wet or dirty feet, or just rolled in a dead rat, now is the time to exercise a little tough love as the new puppy will most likely not want to be alone in their kennel and will prefer sleeping next to you.

If your bed is large enough to accommodate their kennel, this is the best way to help your puppy have a happy sleep time because they will be next to you, but still inside their own kennel, and as they grow larger they will be used to their kennel and will not mind that it is sitting on the floor. Congratulations! You've just created a routine that will ensure happy and respectful sleeping patterns for your dog.

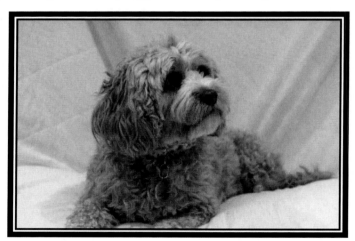

Happy Puppy Play

Taking the time for regular play sessions with your new Cavapoo puppy will certainly make them very happy, so make sure you set aside several times during your day when you stop with the human work and chores and engage your puppy in fun games for 10 or 15 minutes at least three or four times a day.

Every puppy and dog needs some time in their day where they can relax and play a fun game, and this is the beginning of trust and respect between you and your fur friend.

Happy Puppy Housetraining

One of the very first things your new Cavapoo puppy needs to learn is where the bathroom is, and the more vigilant you are, the fewer "accidents" will occur, which will make both of you much happier.

I taught my Shih Tzu (Boris) to ring a little bell whenever he needed to go outside, which is a very valuable "trick" to teach. Just hang a loud ringing bell at the end of a ribbon, string or rope from the doorknob where you will always take your dog through to go outside for a bathroom break. Every time you take them out, go to the bell, lift their paw knock it against the bell to make it ring. Say *"Good boy, or girl – go pee?"* Then immediately take them out through this door.

Learn to pay attention and understand your dog's body language, so that you can help teach them proper bathroom habits at a very young age. This is a smart dog and it should not be difficult to quickly train them that outside is where they need to go to get to their bathroom.

When they wake up in the morning, take them outside immediately. Twenty minutes after they have eaten a meal, take them outside to relieve themselves. After a play session or when they've had a big drink of water, or woken up from a nap, take them outside. After they've gone pee or number 2, immediately praise and reward them with a treat.

Yes, to do this right, you and your puppy will be spending a lot of time going outside, but once their bladder grows larger and stronger, the number of hours he or she can "hold" it will increase, and the number of times your dog will have to visit the great outdoor bathroom during each day will markedly decrease.

Use this bathroom training time also as a way to create a strong bond between you and your dog and as their first lessons in leash training and reward training for doing what you ask; if you take the time to go out with them while they're on leash, it's easy to train your dog to "go" on command, and as they mature, you'll be very glad that you took the time to do this.

Happy Puppy Feeding

It's not rocket science to understand that providing your puppy or dog with the best nutrition from the very first day you bring them home will lead to a healthier fur friend, which in turn, will lead to a feel-good, energetic and happy companion.

Be aware of the importance of what you feed your dog and commit to doing the best you can to keep your canine friend healthy and happy. Read labels and feed them only the highest-quality food, so they have the best opportunity for a long life.

While it's important to start your puppy off with the right food, it's just as important to continue to feed your adult dog the very best diet. Please refer to Chapter 7 (Feeding the Happy Cavapoo), where you will read about types of food, appropriate treats and more.

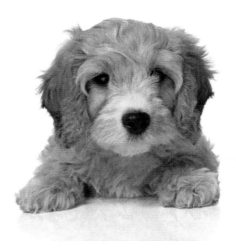

Happy Socializing

Socializing a new puppy is one of the most important steps you can take to ensure that your chosen companion lives a happy and stress-free life.

When you don't take the time to properly socialize your Cavapoo puppy, and indeed, keep on socializing throughout their lifetime, you can actually create many behavioral issues; some of these can be so severe that your dog may be in danger of having their life prematurely shortened, or having to wear a muzzle every time they are in public, should they act out aggressively toward a human or other animal.

Many times, I've been called upon to help a human alleviate aggressive tendencies being displayed by their canine companion, and in pretty much every instance, this could have been entirely avoided if the dog had been properly trained and socialized.

In the case of the adorable Cavapoo, because they are a small breed that is relatively easy to carry around, if you make the mistake of coddling and babying this companion, you can end up creating an insecure dog, or worse, one that is downright disagreeable, with a penchant for acting out toward anyone who gets too close.

Every dog must have a leader. While the charming, loving and playful Cavapoo is usually friendly and peaceful with everyone, every dog can learn to have a stubborn streak. When not properly socialized, trained and taught to respect the word of their human guardians, even this small, sturdy companion may be forced to take over the family "pack" and make human decisions. Unfortunately, this can get them and you into all sorts of unwanted troubles, especially should they decide to act out in an aggressive manner.

Any sort of aggression (while not usually a trait seen in the Cavapoo) is a huge stress on both dog and human and, as we are all aware, stress shortens lives and prevents anyone from experiencing happiness, so help make your dog happy and make sure that you don't place the very heavy burden of making human decisions on the shoulders of your canine companion.

While early socialization of a puppy is very important, keep in mind that it's just as important to continue your adult dog's socialization throughout their lifetime. Please refer to Chapter 10 (Humans Make a LOT of Stupid Mistakes) that outlines the many aspects of socializing your Cavapoo.

Happy Training

Almost as important as proper socializing to keep your dog happy, is proper training, which should never be overlooked, unless you want to create an unstable Cavapoo that barks and growls at everything and thinks they are the boss of all they survey.

This sweet-natured companion breed can be surprisingly versatile and able to excel at sports you may never think to consider, so long as they can be with you, and you have the time and patience to teach. Just because the Cavapoo is designed to be a true companion, doesn't mean that he or she is less capable than their larger counterparts.

Don't be fooled by their smaller stature, because in order to keep any dog happy, they need to have both their body regularly exercised and their brain regularly challenged.

Start training this dog as soon as you bring him or her home from the breeder and you will have given yourself the best opportunity to have a happy, eager to comply and safe companion at your side before they are six months old. Of course, you will start out with very short training sessions of no more than a few minutes at a time, and as they slowly mature, you can increase the length of your sessions.

Make sure any training is a fun and happy time for both you and your dog, with lots of happy praise and treats, and he or she will quickly learn to trust and respect you as their leader and be eager for their next session.

While this puppy can begin training at an early age, when you continue their training throughout their life, this smart and affectionate companion will usually be an eager participant that is entirely capable of learning many commands, tricks, and hand signals, as well as several canine sports. See more in Chapter 12 (Training Basics for a Happy Cavapoo).

Happy Exercising

While the Cavapoo can certainly excel with training and learning new routines, which is exercise as well, they also need some down time, or some time off from your vigilant supervision.

Just like us humans, who need time where they don't have to think about work, our dogs also need some free time where they can enjoy romping and playing with the family or exploring the local woodland paths, rolling in the grass or lazing in the warm sunshine, and just being a dog.

While the Cavapoo can be a moderate-energy dog, depending on their age, they can also be a much higher energy companion, with a playful temperament that loves to chase and romp with other similar sized dogs.

Of course, with a smaller dog, your supervision of playtime is always a must, because allowing a smaller dog to play with a bigger and much heavier dog can mean that your Cavapoo inadvertently gets injured. Supervision is even more important when your Cavapoo gets older and is not as spry as they once were.

While every dog is different, with respect to how much exercise they might need, and how active YOU are will also have an effect, the Cavapoo usually requires a moderate amount of daily exercise to keep them mentally healthy and physically fit. You can learn much more about the exercises that will keep this dog happy in Chapter 6 (Every Happy Cavapoo Wants Exercise).

Happy Visits to the Vet

Even though you may be feeding the best food, properly exercising, socializing and training your dog to be a calm and obedient member of your family, you will also want to have at least yearly visits to your chosen veterinarian's office to make sure all is well.

Start taking your dog to the vet's office even when they don't have any reason to be there, other than to receive a treat and friendly greetings, so that they get used to the different smells and people who work there because when you do this, your dog will learn that visits to the vet's office can be a happy time.

While it's ideal to get your puppy used to visits to the vet's office when they are still young, there is much you can do throughout the life of your adult dog that will help to keep these visits to a minimum. Be sure to read Chapter 8 (Care of the Happy Cavapoo) that outlines many things you can do to help ensure your dog remains as healthy as possible.

Back to the pen and paper exercise.

When you pay attention, and take the time to think about the many things you can do that will keep your dog happy, even more ideas will present themselves along the way, and you and your chosen canine companion will enjoy a long and happy life together. Take my word for it, and *do make the time for this fun exercise* because you will thank me later.

In a Nutshell

The above paragraphs are a short synopsis of what I think makes for a Happy Cavapoo, and I'm sure you may have many more ideas to contribute to this list.

The following Chapters of this book contain much more detail concerning what every conscientious Cavapoo guardian needs to commit to, on a daily basis, in order to ensure that the human family and the chosen canine companion have the best opportunity for living a long, happy and healthy life together without ever having to experience any unwanted behavioral issues.

When you want to raise a Happy Cavapoo canine companion that is a joy to share your life with, you will want to carefully read through all the coming Chapters, while always keeping in mind, not just what makes you and your family happy, but what makes your dog happy as well.

Chapter 3: Overview of the Happy Cavapoo

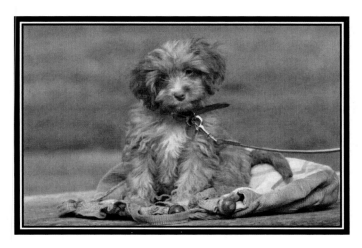

"If I could be half the person my dog is,
I'd be twice the human I am."
— Charles Yu

I cannot stress enough how important it is that you understand the basics of any breed, such as size, energy level, intelligence, temperament, and exercise requirements, so that you can truly understand if you are the right person or family for sharing your life with a particular dog.

In the case of the highly trainable Cavapoo, this means gaining some basic knowledge of the history of this smaller member of the hybrid companion canines.

Learning about the temperament, health and where this dog's parents (the Cavalier King Charles Spaniel and the Miniature Poodle) originally came from will help you choose wisely to ensure that your lifestyle and daily routine can meet this dog's needs.

Cavalier King Charles Spaniel Parent

History: a native of the United Kingdom, historians theorize that during the early part of the 18th century, the red and white version of the

King Charles hunting spaniel was originally known as the "Blenheim", named after the 1st Duke of Marlborough (John Churchill), and that these dogs were bred to keep up with the trotting pace of a horse.

It is believed that divergence from the King Charles Spaniel and the original development of the Cavalier occurred during the turn of the 20th century by using the Toy Trawler Spaniel (now extinct), believed to have descended from the curly-coated King Charles and Sussex spaniels that were originally sporting dogs before they became toy show dogs.

It is also believed that the Cavalier came into existence through the cross breeding of smaller spaniels with the shorter nosed Pug and the Japanese Chin, and that this dog made its way to Scotland during the 1600's, where this spaniel became a fashionable lap dog for the noble class.

These early toy spaniels were quite commonly seen as ladies' companions, and during King Charles II reign (1630 to 1685), this dog was given its royal title of King Charles Spaniel after King Charles II, who was obsessed with his Cavaliers to the point of ignoring important issues of his kingdom. Charles put a law in place declaring that no King Charles Spaniel could be barred from any public place, including where animals otherwise were forbidden, which is still in place today!

Apparently, when serious show dog breeding became popular in England, breeders altered the dog's facial structure so that it would look more like the Pug until an American (Roswell Eldridge) shocked everyone by offering a cash prize at the famous Crufts Dog Show for anyone presenting a dog that resembled those found in early paintings.

After careful breeding, the shorter-faced dogs became the English Toy Spaniel, and those that more closely resembled the original toy spaniels became known as the Cavalier.

As is the case with many breed lines, the Second World War created a serious setback in the creation of this emerging breed with breeding stock at the most well-known kennel (Ttiweh Cavalier Kennel) dropping from 60 to just three, and those that survived the war formed the basis from which all of today's Cavaliers are descended.

It was not until 1956 that the first Cavalier was seen in the United States when Lyon Brown and Elizabeth Spalding imported this spaniel and founded the first US club.

Recently, a team of scientists declared that this toy spaniel is both physically and characteristically the furthest removed from the wolf. This spaniel displays only two of the nine aggressive behaviour patterns and none of the six submissive ones found in the wolf. Apparently, this loving toy spaniel never matures past the age of a 20-day-old wolf puppy for its entire life and remains in a *"neotenic"* state (Peter Pan mode) for his or her lifetime.

Temperament: the affectionate *"Cavalier King Charles Spaniel"* is a sweet-natured, purebred sporting dog that is a member of the Toy Dog category.

This toy spaniel breed is best suited for families that have plenty of time to spend with this playful and eager to please, comfort loving canine companion. This means spending almost all of your day in their presence. If left alone, they will suffer greatly and will usually whine, bark and engage in destructive chewing.

Don't be mislead by this dog's soft and affectionate temperament, because they were once a hunting spaniel and as a result, even though they love to cuddle on the couch, this is also still a sturdy and active dog that will enjoy plenty of outdoor exercise and may chase other small animals.

Patient, gentle and friendly with their children and the rest of their family, the Cavalier is also usually accepting of all other pets in their flock, whether furred, feathered or human. However, when not properly socialized from an early age, this spaniel can become wary, timid and nervous, which may lead to fearful aggressiveness toward unknown dogs, other pets or humans.

This affectionate, non-threatening spaniel can be the perfect companion for seniors, first-time dog guardians and nervous smaller children, because they are always patient, happy, and willing to play.

As a result of this dog's friendly and trusting nature, while they may bark when visitors or thieves arrive, he or she will be a poor watchdog (and an even worse guard dog), as they will happily welcome all comers, and show them where the valuables are kept.

This loving breed will become very attached and devoted to its family members and if you neglect him or her and do not provide them with regular daily exercise and mental stimulation, they may create their own entertainment through destructive behavior.

Recognized by the American Kennel Club (AKC) in 1995, the elegant and charming Cavalier King Charles Spaniel is a friendly dog with a soft temperament that currently holds the #18 popularity position amongst the 192 registered purebreds.

Be aware that this dog can develop many serious health issues, which may lead to a shortened lifespan.

Miniature Poodle Parent

History: the Poodle has been known throughout Western Europe for 400 years or more. Many falsely believe that this breed originated in France, because they are often referred to as the *"French Poodle"*. However, this purebred canine was originally a working dog bred and developed in both Germany and Russia for field hunting, which involved retrieving downed waterfowl in the water.

While still other claims of Poodle origin have been attributed to Denmark and the ancient Piedmont in Northern Mesopotamia, one thing that is certain is that today's modern Poodle was a descendant of the now-extinct French Water Dog, the Barbet, and possibly the Hungarian Water Hound.

Believed to be one of the oldest hunting breeds used for water retrieval, this dog is referred to as the *"French Poodle"*, because the breed was standardized in France where it then became the national dog of this country.

What many people don't realize is that the Poodle may be one of the oldest breeds of canines known to man, having appeared on ancient

Greek and Roman coins during the time of Emperor Augustus, as long ago as 30 A.D.

As well, the Poodle was revered in pictures that were carved on many monuments, tombs and palace walls and there is historic evidence of the intelligent Poodle seen in medieval manuscripts of the 15th, 16th and 17th centuries.

As the Poodle became well known as a distinct breed, they were bred down in size to become more of a companion dog, which resulted in the creation of the Miniature and Toy sizes of the breed.

Despite the Poodle's origins as a hunting and retrieving breed, they became well known for their abilities as performing dogs, and were widely distributed due largely to traveling gypsies who favored the Poodle above all others as a performing circus dog.

With careful breeding practices, the off square body shape began to change to increase their ability for faster agility, which was not possible with the longer retriever body shape. This resulted in the Poodle becoming more of a square shape to improve the dogs' spinning and hind leg acrobatic capabilities.

Interestingly, the standard, more square shape of all sizes of the Poodle breed is a result of improving their abilities as performing circus dogs, rather than as a hunting or retrieving breed, which makes the intelligent Poodle a multi-talented purebred canine.

While other breeds were agile and intelligent, what the Poodle had that all others did not, was their comical and striking appearance and hair that could be cut into different shapes and even colored and fashioned to resemble a clown's attire. It was this unique combination that made the Poodle such an eye-catching, charismatic entertainer.

During the 18th century smaller poodles became popular with royals and thus the three official sizes of this popular purebred became the Toy, Miniature and Standard Poodle.

Interestingly, the Poodle did not receive great popularity until after World War II, at which time this intelligent canine quickly became the canine of choice and as such enjoyed being the most popular dog in America for over 20 years.

Temperament: the Miniature Poodle has a delightful, loving temperament, often described as alert, active, faithful, highly intelligent, and easily trainable.

This dog is not a breed particularly well suited for the elderly or for humans that lead busy lives with long work schedules that keep them away from home. In order for the Miniature Poodle to be well balanced psychologically, they demand a lot of attention and will not be happy spending only a few minutes with their humans each day.

While some breeds of dogs of lower intelligence might be just fine without receiving daily interesting activities to keep them busy and mentally challenged, the Miniature Poodle (with their lively and playful temperament) typically wants and needs to occupy much more of their guardian's time and energy by engaging in physical activities that also challenge them mentally.

A Miniature Poodle guardian will need to constantly be thinking of ways to challenge their bright and inquisitive canine companion and make their daily life interesting. Otherwise, this intelligent dog may think of ways to entertain themselves that could involve destroying the contents of your home or engaging in non-stop barking to vocalize their unhappiness.

This will be a loyal and loving dog that will bond very quickly with any and all family members in a very short period of time. This is a dog that loves being loved, which means that it is very easy for them to be heartbroken when their owners leave them alone.

While the Miniature Poodle is usually shy around strangers, they rarely act aggressively, and will get along well with other animals in the home, so long as they are slowly and properly introduced to them. This dog is an enormous people pleaser, who absolutely loves to perform and show off their skills, this fur friend will thrive on positive praise and physical affection.

If there is tension in your home, with angry, raised voices or emotional humans that often get into disagreements or fights, the Poodle is not a good choice for you. This sensitive breed is easily upset by loud arguments and stress energy. Any type of disharmonious home life can literally cause this dog to manifest digestive upsets and neurotic behaviors that can make them literally sick to their stomachs.

NOTE: the very sensitive Miniature Poodle will not be good with small children who tend to be unpredictable, loud and boisterous. Also note that some Miniature Poodle breeding lines have become too high-strung and nervous, and this is where you will find those hypersensitive and neurotic Poodles that give the rest of the breed a bad name.

Even though much of a Poodle's personality will depend upon how well they are socialized as puppies and what sort of ongoing training they receive, keep in mind that this companion is a peaceful, sensitive dog that needs a peaceful, harmonious home life.

First recognized by the American Kennel Club in 1886, the very popular Poodle continues to be one of the most popular dog breed worldwide, having remained amongst the top 10 favorites out of 192 registered breeds for many years in a row.

OK, now you have a basic understanding of the history and temperament of both of the Cavapoo's breed parents, what does this mean for the Cavapoo hybrid?

Following is the main overview of the breed, which will be the foundation of choosing a Cavapoo wisely and raising a happy and well-behaved dog.

Cavapoo Vital Statistics

While every dog is unique, there are standards that are common to each purebred canine, such as height, weight and various coat colors and features. You can also get a pretty good idea of what the puppies will look like when full grown, when you see their parents.

Height and Weight

When measured at the shoulder, the Cavapoo may stand between 9 and 14 inches (23 and 36 centimetres) and ideally weigh between 12 and 25 pounds (5 and 11 kilograms) or more, depending on the size of both breed parents, with an average lifespan of between 10 and 15 years, with many living even longer.

Coat Colors and Common Features

This small and popular designer breed has a sturdy body, strong legs, a dark nose, medium length pendant ears, and a loving, friendly and playful disposition.

The soft coat of the Cavapoo will usually be curly or wavy, depending on which parent genes are more dominant. Coat color can vary widely and will include apricot, black, brown, chestnut, cream, red sable, sable, white, tri-color (black, tan and white) or other variations of colors.

Eyes will be large, round and dark in color with a friendly, trusting expression and when they are happy the tail will be carried level or with a slight upward curve.

How Smart is the Cavapoo?

While every dog is surprisingly different even within the same breed, despite what some "experts" might have to say about it, you need to keep in mind that there are *"people smarts"* and *"dog smarts"* and that these two ways of rating intelligence are often widely divergent or in conflict with one another.

If you really want to rate your Cavapoo's intelligence, based on what we humans think is *"smart",* there is a book *("The Intelligence of Dogs")* written in 1994 by Stanley Coren, which has become the standard for rating the particular intelligence of different canine breeds.

While I can agree, in part, with some of the information contained in this book, I can also disagree. I have much personal experience with many breeds, and have found that some dogs that are rated very low on the intelligence scale are also very smart in their own way.

Therefore, I caution you not to pre-handicap your dog's level of intelligence just because of something you may have read in a well-respected book, because each dog has their own unique set of talents and much of how they develop mentally is up to their guardian.

With respect to the Cavapoo, we need to look at the intelligence level of both breed parents to get a good idea of how smart the offspring will usually be.

Coren judges canine intelligence of particular purebred canines based on three categories, as follows:

*"**Instinctive Intelligence** – a dog's ability to carry out tasks it was bred to perform, such as guarding, herding, hunting, pointing, retrieving or supplying companionship."*

*"**Adaptive Intelligence** – how well a dog is able to solve problems on its own."*

*"**Working/Obedience Intelligence** – how quickly a dog is able to learn from humans."*

In the case of the Cavapoo's breed parents, Coren places the Cavalier in the *"Average Working/Obedience Intelligence"* category, and the Poodle in the *"Brightest Dogs"* category. This means that the Cavapoo offspring will very likely be highly intelligent, willing to please and easy to train.

Please keep in mind that there are always exceptions to every study and a particular breed's degree of intelligence is often related to their early upbringing and how they are trained.

I have had considerable personal experience with this breed, and can tell you that they are eager to learn and very easy to train, even though they can sometimes have a bit of a stubborn streak, and because they can be sensitive, will not respond well to harsh training, which means that you will have to be patient and find just the right tone when working with this dog.

There is no doubt that with the proper training method and plenty of calm consistency, the Cavapoo is easily trainable, and they will be happy and mentally fit so long as they are permitted to spend most of their time in the company of their human guardians.

Temperament of the Cavapoo

Whether your devoted Cavapoo is energetic or tends toward being a more laid back and snuggly lap dog, they are certainly going to be an affectionate, playful, happy dog that bonds strongly to humans of all ages, and truly loves everyone they meet along their exciting road of life.

Every dog needs the discipline of being regularly walked on leash outside of the home each day, as well as the opportunity for off-leash time to run and play fetch or enjoy socializing with other dogs.

Although the temperament of a Cavapoo (or any dog) will vary from dog to dog, and be somewhat dependent upon their first weeks with the breeder, as well as the human guardian who has trained and socialized them during the first few months of their life, generally speaking, this breed displays a loyal and affectionate personality with an alert, outgoing and social temperament.

Proper socializing and teaching basic commands should begin at a young age for the Cavapoo, who can begin to learn basic commands at ten weeks of age.

The Cavapoo is an intelligent, highly trainable hybrid canine created to be a companion lap dog, with the purpose of providing love and companionship to their human family. This means that while they prefer to be close to their human guardians at all times, they have a kind, friendly and outgoing nature. This is a sweet, obedient dog that usually gets along favourably with everyone, including children, unknown adults, other dogs and animals.

This little charmer will generally be an eager to please quick learner that loves to perform and learn new things, so long as you teach with fun and kindness and provide him or her with plenty of praise and tasty treats as rewards for a job well done.

Always keep in mind that any dog, including the Cavapoo, can become snappish if teased, provoked or feeling that it must protect itself. Therefore, a guardian should always be watchful when their dog is in the presence of younger children or feeling nervous around much larger dogs.

Generally speaking, the Cavapoo is a small, sturdy, adaptable and versatile little dog that is just as happy going for a long walk with you as they will be learning tricks, running an Agility course, going on a road trip or sitting quietly beside you (or on your lap), while you watch a movie.

The adult Cavapoo is certainly capable of excelling at several canine sports, such as Agility, Flyball, Trick Training, Advanced Obedience and more. Further, when properly trained and socialized this dog also has the personality to brighten the days of many people as a wonderful therapy dog.

Whatever you teach this dog, at a minimum, make sure that you always get them outside for several, daily, 30-40 minute walks and allow them some off-leash time to run and sniff or play with other small dogs.

The highest priority for a Cavapoo is always that they be allowed to be part of whatever the family is enjoying, and because they are quite sturdy for their small size, they can be very good companions for children who are old enough to understand how to respect a dog.

This breed will become very attached and devoted to its family members, and they will not usually be aggressive toward strangers or other dogs unless they have not been properly socialized at a young age.

This is an affectionate, often energetic, playful dog that needs daily exercising as well as mental stimulation in order to remain healthy. If you neglect this dog and do not ensure that their needs are met, they may create their own entertainment, which could include barking to excess.

The Cavapoo will be a good family dog that is affectionate and totally devoted and while they may not be a particularly good guard dog because they are very friendly to almost everyone, they will be good watch dogs who will alert you when someone is approaching.

When they are puppies, it's important to engage them in thinking and working activities because they need this stimulation as part of their on-going healthy development.

Just keep in mind that how active you are will likely have a sizeable impact on the health of your Cavapoo who will need to eliminate pent up energy by exercising their minds and their bodies so that they can remain a healthy weight.

All puppies are energetic, including the Cavapoo puppy, and if you are active with them at a young age, and engage them in training and activities that stretch their minds and bodies, chances are that they will continue to be active into their adult years. On the other hand, if you are an inactive human, the chances are high that your dog will become overweight, which can shorten their life.

Bottom line with this breed is that while the Cavapoo can certainly defend his or herself if pushed too far, they are rarely aggressive, and only if not socialized, or backed into a corner they can see no way out of. This means that this small companion can be a good choice for families with children, especially since they are playful and sturdy enough to play without coming to harm.

This is a dog that craves human companionship and will be happiest spending a good part of his or her day being your constant shadow and, depending on the activity level of their human guardian, they will be playful and energetic or less active, often enjoying spending time snoozing next to you.

Special Needs

The Cavapoo hybrid dog has been created to provide companionship and all the comforts that an indoor lifestyle provides. In other words, this is not a dog to be left alone in a back yard. They are simply not designed to withstand extremes of temperature or being left alone. As well, forcing this companion to spend many hours alone each day could cause them to become nervous or develop separation anxiety.

The Cavapoo is too small to be able to effectively protect his or herself against the attack of a larger dog. As well, depending on their adult size, and especially when they are still puppies, they can be prey to large hunting birds, such as owls, hawks and eagles that could swoop down into a yard and carry them off.

Happy Cavapoo secrets

The name *"Cavapoo"* is a meshing together of the first few letters of each breed parent (**Cava**lier King Charles Spaniel and **Poo**dle).

The Cavapoo may also be known as the *"Cavoodle"* or "Cavadoodle".

As a result of their affectionate, sweet nature, the Cavapoo can easily excel as a therapy dog.

In a Nutshell

Familiarizing yourself with the Cavapoo's size, weight, special needs, and early history and what they were originally developed to do, plus understanding their intelligence level, temperament and exercise requirements will help you to decide if the hybrid Cavapoo is the right dog for you and your family.

Obtaining a comprehensive understanding of the breed's needs will not only save you and your dog from much future grief, but it will be a pre-requisite for raising a content, well-behaved, and happy dog that you are proud to call your best friend and companion.

Chapter 4: Healthy Cavapoo = Happy Dog

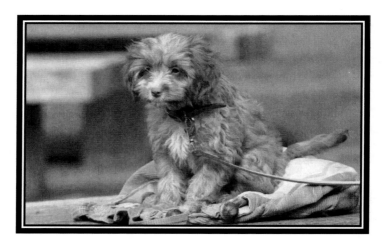

"Dogs are not our whole life,
but they make our lives whole."
— Roger Caras

If your Cavapoo is not physically healthy, he or she will not be a happy canine companion for very long, because suffering from health-related issues can easily create a miserable and ill-mannered dog.

It's prudent that you take the many steps outlined here to help ensure that you are doing all that you can to keep on top of your Cavapoo's good health.

Make sure you take the time to choose a veterinarian that can provide yearly check-ups, have your dog spayed or neutered in a timely fashion, choose a healthy diet for him or her, and carefully read this section so that you educate yourself about issues that may adversely affect your dog's health.

As well, take the time to learn a little canine CPR, because doing so may save the life of your own dog, or someone else's.

Below you will find more information on each one of these steps you need to take to raise a healthy and happy Cavapoo.

Choose your veterinarian wisely

Some clinics specialize in caring for smaller pets, while some specialize in larger animal care, and others have a wide-ranging area of expertise and will care for all animals, including livestock and reptiles.

Choosing a good veterinary clinic will be very similar to choosing the right health care clinic or doctor for your own personal health, because you want to ensure that your puppy or adult dog receives the quality care they deserve. A good place to begin your search will be by asking other dog owners where they take their furry friends and whether they are happy with the service they receive.

It's also a good idea to take your Cavapoo into your chosen clinic several times before they actually need to be there for any treatment, so that they are not fearful of the new smells and unfamiliar surroundings.

Consider timely neutering or spaying

There are varying opinions on the topic of the best time to neuter or spay your young Cavapoo. One thing that most veterinarians do agree on is that earlier spaying or neutering, between 4 and 6 months of age, can be a better choice than waiting longer.

Keep in mind that non-neutered or spayed males and females are more likely to display aggression related to sexual behaviour, than are dogs that have been neutered or spayed.

For instance, fighting, particularly in male dogs that is directed at other males, is less common after neutering. The intensity of other types of aggression, such as irritable aggression in females will be totally eliminated by spaying, so make that appointment at the vet's office and get it done.

Effects on General Temperament: many dog owners often become needlessly worried that a neutered or spayed dog will lose their vigor, when in fact, many unwanted, aggressive qualities, resulting from hormonal impact, may resolve after surgery, and you will be acting as a conscientious, informed, and caring guardian.

Effects on Escape and Roaming: a neutered or spayed Cavapoo is less likely to wander, and castrated male dogs have the tendency to patrol smaller sized outdoor areas and are less likely to participate in territorial conflicts with perceived opponents.

Possible Weight Gain: while metabolic changes that occur after spaying or neutering can cause some puppies to gain weight, often the real culprit for any weight gain is the human who feels guilty for subjecting their puppy to this medical procedure, and in an attempt to make themselves feel better, they feed more treats or meals to their companion.

If you notice weight gain after neutering or spaying your Cavapoo puppy, simply adjust their food and treat consumption as needed and once stitches are healed, make sure that they are receiving adequate daily exercise.

Educate yourself with respect to vaccination

It has now become common practice to vaccinate adult dogs every three years, and if your veterinarian is insisting on a yearly vaccination for your puppy, you need to ask them why, because to do otherwise is considered by many professionals to be *"over vaccinating"*.

Whether or not your dog actually needs a booster can be determined with a simple blood test at your vet's office, so be proactive, and ask for a blood test.

Puppies need to be vaccinated in order to provide them with protection against four common and serious diseases referred to as *"DAPP"*, which stands for Distemper, Adenovirus, Parainfluenza and Parvo Virus.

Approximately one week after your puppy has completed all three sets of primary DAPP vaccinations, they will be fully protected from those specific diseases.

Be aware of the health conditions that may affect your dog

A healthy, happy Cavapoo may live to be 15 years or more, and with healthy breeding practices and proper care may not suffer from any noted health problems.

However, this hybrid canine is half Cavalier King Charles Spaniel, and half Miniature Poodle. In other words, we need to consider the health problems that may commonly affect both of these purebreds, and then especially take note of problems that may affect both breeds.

Cavalier King Charles Spaniel Health Problems

While a healthy Cavalier King Charles Spaniel may live to be 9 to 14 years (more or less), and with proper care they may not suffer from any of the below noted health concerns, it is prudent to list all concerns possibly associated with this breed so that you have a clear understanding of problems that *"may"* affect your dog, including:

Hip Dysplasia: is caused when the head of the dog's femur does not fit properly into the hip joint socket. Factors that have an influence include nutrition, a dog's environment and the condition of the hips of its parents. Screening for hip dysplasia is recommended for breeding stock.

Patellar Luxation: this slipping kneecap condition is a common defect seen in many breeds that may also be caused by accidentally falling or jumping from a height. Often, you will see a dog with this problem appear to be skipping down the road as they occasionally lift one leg when the kneecap slips out of the patellar groove and the leg locks up.

Surgery is the treatment option for this condition, although many dogs live a relatively normal life with this defect.

Entropion: is a condition in which the dog's eyelid will roll inward which then causes the lashes to rub against the eyeball. Left untreated, this condition can severely damage the dog's eye, even causing blindness. Surgery is required to correct this problem.

Cataracts: usually appear between the ages of two and four years and are common in many breeds. This is an eye condition where the lens becomes cloudy or milky, which would be like trying to see through a foggy window. This eye condition can also appear in juveniles from birth to 3 years of age and will usually lead to blindness.

Progressive Retinal Atrophy (PRA): causes degeneration of the retina, which is part of the eye. The retina is the part that senses visual information and sends it to the brain. Degeneration of this vital part of the eye eventually will lead to blindness and this disease usually appears between 3 and 5 years of age. A simple DNA test is available to determine (without waiting for symptoms to appear).

Corneal Dystrophy: this disease is a change in the eye usually attributed to aging, causing fluid leakage that appears as a bluish color in the inner layer of the cornea.

Distichiasis: is an eye problem where an eyelash grows in an abnormal location in the dog's eyelid. This is often caused when multiple eyelashes grow from a single duct and this problem can affect both upper and lower eyelids even though a dog's lower lids usually have no eyelashes. A problem eyelash can cause irritation, squinting, and redness and if left untreated can scar the cornea of the dog's eye. Treatment involves removal of the offending lash or lashes.

Keratoconjunctivitis Sicca (KCS): is a common disease defined as a reduction of natural tear production, occurring as a result of inflammation and an increase in mucous discharge, which is often misdiagnosed as bacterial conjunctivitis. While traditional treatment involves replacement of diminished tears, there is a relatively new immunosuppressant eye drop treatment (Cyclosporine A) that has proven to be therapeutic.

Syringomyelia (SM): is a non-contagious inherited condition caused by conformation rather than a disease, that occurs when a fluid-filled sac develops on the dog's spinal cord, caused by malformation of the bones of the skull and the brain.

Much more likely to occur in small dogs as a result of their smaller skull size, it is a chronic and progressively degenerative condition often causing intense pain and headaches. Other symptoms can include stiffness and numbness of the dog's neck, back and legs, as well as loss of bladder and bowel control or the inability to regulate body temperature. Treatment involves surgery and various medications to reduce pain, swelling and fluid production.

Deafness (Inherited): inherited deafness affects quite a number of dog breeds and in most cases is associated with white coat coloration around the head, as this is linked to the piebald and/or merle genes. Deafness usually occurs in puppies within a few weeks of birth and it can occur in only one ear, or both ears. There is no cure and puppies that are deaf in both ears are often euthanized because they are accident prone, startle easily, which can lead to biting, and they can be difficult to train.

Primary Secretory Otitis Media (PSOM): this ear problem affects almost half of the Cavalier breed and is also known as "glue ear" because it can cause a severe mucus plug in the dog's middle ear, which can cause the tympanic membrane to bulge.

Epilepsy: is considered a neurological problem. While the most common cause of seizures is idiopathic epilepsy, which is an inherited form of epilepsy, they can be caused by many factors, including physical trauma, such as a head injury. If seizures begin, it will be very important to have your dog diagnosed.

Thrombocytopenia: is a bleeding disorder that could be life threatening, in which the platelets (fragments of cells) are insufficient in number to form a plug around an injured area to stop bleeding. Signs of a dog suffering from this condition may include tiredness, weakness, loss of appetite, small hemorrhages inside the mouth or under the skin (stomach and groin area), nosebleeds, blood in the urine or prolonged bleeding after surgery or an injury.

Treatment will depend upon the underlying cause and severity and if platelet levels are very low, blood transfusions may be necessary. If there is infection, antibiotics would be prescribed and treatment may involve the use of corticosteroids or other immune suppressing drugs.

Weakened Immune System: can result in various disorders, such as allergies, dry eye, cancers, muscle and nerve problems, thyroid and blood problems or digestive and metabolic problems.

Heart Murmurs or Arrhythmia: while an occasional irregular sounding heart beat may not be a concern or cause other more serious problems, this may be an early symptom of an underlying condition, that could be more serious, which means that it would be wise to have your veterinarian check it out.

Mitral Valve Disease (MVD): is a degeneration of the mitral heart valve that can lead to heart failure. If a dog has this problem, the blood will flow back into the chamber, which can cause the chamber to enlarge, which then can cause other problems, including an irregular heartbeat, constricted windpipe or flowing back into the lungs.

The first sign of mitral valve disease is a heart murmur, which can usually only be heard with a stethoscope. Symptoms include fainting, coughing, increased blood pressure, tiredness and reluctance to exercise. There is no cure and beyond replacing the valve, management involves various drug therapies to improve the dog's quality of life.

Obesity: is one of the most common and preventable health hazards. It is not often considered when deciding to share your life with a canine companion that most dogs are active athletes. This means that if you do not provide your dog with the opportunity to exercise in a way that is optimal for their size and weight, you will have a fat dog.

Many dogs are overweight, simply because they love to eat and when love of eating is combined with little or no exercise, this leads to laziness and obesity. While obesity is a serious condition that plagues many breeds of dogs, the Cavalier seems to be more prone to this health problem. When they do not receive sufficient daily exercise, they will quickly become overweight, which can create or exacerbate other health problems.

Miniature Poodle Health Problems

While a healthy Miniature Poodle may live to be 10 to 18 years (more or less), and with proper care they may not suffer from any of the below noted health concerns, it is prudent to list all concerns possibly associated with this breed so that you have a clear understanding of problems that *"may"* affect your dog, including:

Progressive Retinal Atrophy (PRA): causes degeneration of the retina, which is part of the eye. The retina is the part that senses visual information and sends it to the brain. Degeneration of this vital part of the eye eventually will lead to blindness and this disease usually appears between 3 and 5 years of age. A simple DNA test is available to determine (without waiting for symptoms to appear).

Cataracts: can appear from birth to 3 years old and usually lead to blindness. Cataracts appearing after age three are usually milder.

Glaucoma: this eye disease, which is usually caused by an increase of fluid pressure in the eye, can cause permanent damage to the dog's vision in the affected eye or eyes, which, if left untreated, can lead to blindness.

Corneal Ulcers: when the clear outer capsule in the dog's eye becomes irritated, scratched or somehow damaged through injury that is left untreated, the area becomes inflamed and bacteria can enter which can then lead to infection which will then cause an ulcer.

A dog suffering from a scratch or an ulcer on the cornea of the eye will be experiencing pain, tearing and itching and often discharge, and will often squint and paw at the eye, which can make the problem worse. Treatment will depend upon how severe the ulcer may be and while milder cases will involve applying antibiotic ointments, more severe cases can involve surgery.

Ectropion: in a dog suffering from this condition the lower eyelid will turn outward and requires surgery to repair.

Entropion: is a condition in which the dog's eyelid will roll inward which then causes the lashes to rub against the eyeball. Left untreated, this condition can severely damage the dog's eye, even causing blindness. Surgery is required to correct this problem.

Otitis Externa: is an inflammation of the ear canal, which can become chronic, and causes discomfort, irritation and pain. Ear infections are common in Miniature Poodles due to the long narrow ear canals, long ears and profuse hair growth in the ear canals.

Cushing's Disease: there are three forms of Cushing's Disease and most dogs suffer from the more common form, *"Pituitary Dependent PD"*, which is a slow growing form of cancer that is located in the pituitary gland caused by an increase in cortisone as a result of a benign tumor. There are many symptoms including obesity, increased thirst and urination, loss of hair, bruising, lack of energy and excessive panting. Once diagnosed, symptoms will be treated with daily oral medication.

Cancer: Miniature Poodles affected by cancer are often those which were not neutered or spayed. Therefore, if you do not require your poodle to remain sexually intact for breeding, it makes sense to have them neutered or spayed.

Hypothyroidism: is a condition resulting from an inadequate production of thyroid hormone, which is treated with medication. Symptoms include lethargy, obesity, excessive hunger and a coarse coat texture. Testing for thyroid malfunction is done through blood sample.

Dental Disease: as a result of their smaller jaw, the Miniature Poodle is prone to dental disease.

Pancreatitis: is especially common in middle-aged, overweight Miniature Poodles who are pudgy around the middle because they are overfed and/or do not get enough daily exercise. Never suddenly give these dogs a meal or a treat that has a very high fat content, because this is the most common trigger of a pancreatitis attack, which can be fatal.

Obesity: I've seen many overweight Poodles, which is one of the most common and preventable health hazards not often considered when deciding to share your life with a canine companion. Most dogs are active athletes, which means that if you do not provide your dog with the opportunity to exercise in a way that is optimal for their size and weight, you will have a fat dog.

Many dogs are overweight, simply because they love to eat and while your Cavapoo may not be a big eater, if they get little or no exercise, which then leads to laziness, much like us humans, they will easily become obese, which can create or exacerbate other health problems.

When you take good care of your happy Cavapoo's health, and they come from a trusted breeder, he or she may never have to suffer from any of the above-noted list of health problems.

Educate Yourself About Common Canine Diseases and Viruses

While your dog may never suffer from a common disease or virus, in order to ensure the safety and health of your happy Cavapoo, you need to be aware of the many common diseases and viruses that could detrimentally affect the health of your dog.

Always watch out for the symptoms of the following common diseases and if you suspect that your dog has been infected, contact your vet immediately.

Distemper (sometimes called *"hard pad disease"*): is a contagious, serious, and deadly viral illness that is spread through the air or by direct or indirect contact with a dog (or other animal) that is already infected (such as ferrets, raccoons, foxes, skunks and wolves), that can also cause thickening of the pads on the feet or nose.

Early symptoms include fever, loss of appetite and mild eye inflammation that may only last a day or two, with symptoms becoming more serious and noticeable as the disease progresses. There is no known cure.

Adenovirus: causes infectious canine hepatitis, which can range in severity from very mild to very serious. The treatment focuses on management of symptoms, and the condition can sometimes result in death. Symptoms can vary and may include coughing, loss of appetite, increased thirst and urination, tiredness, vomiting and seizures.

Canine Parainfluenza Virus (CPIV): also referred to as *"canine influenza virus"*, *"greyhound disease"* or *"race flu"*, which is easily spread through the air or by coming into contact with respiratory secretions. While it is usually a self-limiting virus that will run its course within a couple of weeks, in severe cases and without antibiotic treatment, it may be fatal.

Symptoms can include a dry, hacking cough, difficulty breathing, wheezing, runny nose and eyes, sneezing, fever, loss of appetite, tiredness, depression and possible pneumonia. In cases where only a cough exists, tests will be required to determine whether the cause of the cough is the parainfluenza virus or the less serious *"kennel cough"*.

Canine Parvovirus (CPV): is a highly contagious viral illness affecting puppies and dogs, foxes, coyotes and wolves. Symptoms include vomiting, bloody diarrhoea, weight loss, and lack of appetite. Without prompt and proper treatment, dogs that have severe parvovirus infections can die within 48 to 72 hours.

Treatment will involve addressing dehydration and correcting electrolyte imbalances by administering intravenous fluids. Anti-inflammatory and antibiotic drugs are also given to control or prevent septicaemia, as well as drugs to control diarrhoea and vomiting.

Other Diseases and Viruses to Be Aware Of

What is Zoonotic? Zoonotic means a contagious disease that can be spread between both animals and humans.

Rabies: is a viral, zoonotic disease transmitted by coming into contact with the saliva of an infected animal, usually through a bite. The virus travels to the brain along the nerves and once symptoms develop (usually marked by a change in temperament), after a prolonged period of suffering, death is almost certainly inevitable. There is no treatment.

In most countries, vaccination against rabies is mandatory between the ages of twelve and sixteen weeks. If you plan to travel out of State or across country borders, you will need to make sure that your dog has an up-to-date Rabies Vaccination Certificate (NASPHV form 51) indicating they have been inoculated against rabies.

Leishmaniasis: is a contagious zoonotic infection caused by a parasite and is transmitted by a bite from a sand fly. While treatment involves the administration of a special drug (sodium stibogluconate), there is no definitive answer for effectively combating Leishmaniasis (especially since one vaccine will not prevent the known multiple species), with the prognosis often being fatal.

Symptoms include loss of appetite, diarrhoea, severe weight loss, exercise intolerance, vomiting, nosebleed, tarry feces, fever, pain in the joints, excessive thirst and urination, inflammation of the muscles, and death from kidney failure.

Lyme Disease: is one of the most common zoonotic tick-borne diseases in the world, which is transmitted by Borrelia bacteria found in the deer or sheep tick. Symptoms of this disease in a young or adult dog include recurrent lameness from joint inflammation, loss of appetite, depression, stiff walk with arched back, sensitivity to touch, swollen lymph nodes, fever, kidney damage, as well as rare heart or nervous system complications.

Control of the symptoms involves a lengthy course of antibiotic treatment in order to completely eliminate the organism.

Rocky Mountain Spotted Fever (RMSF): is a zoonotic disease transmitted by both the American dog tick and the RMSF tick, which must be attached to the dog for a minimum of five hours in order to transmit the disease.

Common symptoms include fever, reduced appetite, depression, painful joints, lameness, vomiting and diarrhoea, and some dogs may develop heart abnormalities, pneumonia, kidney failure, liver damage, or even neurological signs, such as seizures or unsteady, wobbly or stumbling gait. Treatment involves a 2-3 week course of antibiotics (Doxycycline or Tetracycline).

Ehrlichiosis: a tick-borne disease transmitted by both the brown dog tick and the Lone Star Tick, with common symptoms including depression, reduced appetite, fever, stiff and painful joints and bruising. The signs of infection typically occur less than a month after a tick bite and last for approximately four weeks. There is no vaccine available. Treatment involves a long course of antibiotics.

Anaplasmosis: deer ticks and Western blacklegged ticks are carriers of the bacteria that transmit canine Anaplasmosis. However, there is also another form of Anaplasmosis (caused by a different bacteria) that is carried by the brown dog tick.

Because the deer tick also carries other diseases, some animals may be at risk of developing more than one tick-borne disease at the same time. Signs are similar to Ehrlichiosis and include painful joints, diarrhoea, fever, and vomiting, as well as possible nervous system disorders. Treatment involves administering the antibiotic Doxycycline for a 30-day period.

Tick Paralysis: this zoonotic infection is caused when ticks attach themselves to the skin and secrete a neurotoxin that affects the nervous system. Affected dogs show signs of weakness and limpness approximately one week after being first bitten.

Symptoms usually begin with a change in pitch of the dog's usual bark, and weakness in the rear legs that eventually involves all four legs, followed by the dog showing difficulty breathing and swallowing. Your dog can die if not diagnosed and properly treated by removal of the tick.

Canine Coronavirus: this highly contagious intestinal disease, which is spread through the feces of contaminated dogs, while now found worldwide, can be destroyed by most commonly available disinfectants. Symptoms include diarrhoea, vomiting and weight loss or anorexia. There is a vaccine available, which is usually given to puppies, because they are more susceptible at a young age. This vaccine is also given to show dogs that have a higher risk of exposure to the disease.

Leptospirosis: is a worldwide zoonotic bacterial infection that can affect humans and many different kinds of animals, including dogs. If left untreated, there is potential for both dogs and humans to die from this disease.

The good news is that this virus is usually treated with antibiotics and supportive care, and because you can protect your dog with a vaccination, it makes sense to vaccinate against this disease if you and your dog live in an area considered a hot spot for leptospirosis.

<u>Be aware that allergies can adversely affect your dog's health</u>

One of the most common complaints discussed at the veterinarian's office when they see dogs obsessively scratching, biting, licking and chewing at their skin or paws is possible allergies, and there can be many triggers. When you educate yourself, you can help ensure your Cavapoo never has to suffer from allergies and can lead a healthier and happier life.

Environmental allergies: what many of us humans seem to forget is that our dogs can develop allergies to dust, chemicals, grass, mould, pollen, car exhaust, various forms of smoke, or flea and tick preparations, as well as allergies to materials such as wool or cotton, and chemicals found in washing soap or chemicals found in cleaning products you use around your home.

Visual symptoms are usually first noticed on the dog's stomach, inside of their legs, and at their tail or paws. Because many allergies are seasonal, our dogs will often be more affected in the spring or fall, with some airborne irritants inhaled by your dog resulting in coughing, sneezing or watery eyes.

Pay attention and if you think that your dog may have come in contact with an irritant found somewhere in your environment, first give them a cleansing bath, with the proper canine shampoo and conditioner.

Junk food allergies: *"True"* food allergies usually account for only about 10% of allergy problems in our canine friends.

Be aware that itching, chewing and chronic ear infections are not actually caused by food allergies, but rather are the result of a suppressed immune system, which is the result of your dog eating a low-quality diet. Food sensitivity issues can often be completely resolved by changing your dog's diet to a high-quality food that is more easily digested.

For instance, check food ingredients because far too many dog food products contain gluten ingredients that are common allergens to our fur friends, such as corn, wheat and soybeans. Become a label reader and ask questions, before you choose your dog's food.

Take the Time to Learn a Little Canine CPR

Of course, nobody wants to find his or herself in a situation where the life of their precious canine companion is put at risk. However, the reality is that accidents happen, and therefore knowing a little bit about how to help save your beloved furry friend is time well spent.

First of all, remember to handle an injured dog very carefully and gently. A dog that is traumatized, fearful or in pain, even one that is usually gentle, may lash out and try to bite.

Consider taking a class, because there are many animal CPR courses being offered these days through community educational systems or even online.

It's also a good idea to put together a canine first aid kit, both at home and in your vehicle, in case of emergencies, that includes the following items:

- Antiseptic Wash for wounds (hydrogen peroxide)
- Blanket
- Gauze Bandaging
- Kwik Stop styptic powder
- Medical Tape
- Nail Clippers
- Non-Stick Bandages for wounds
- Scissors
- Sterile Eye Wash
- Tick Twister
- Towel
- Tweezers
- Wash cloth

It would also be prudent to obtain a copy of the American Red Cross emergency techniques called *"Saving Your Pet With CPR"*, and familiarize yourself with the proper way to administer CPR to a dog.

Artificial Respiration Step by Step

If your dog becomes unconscious, depending upon what happened to them, they may stop breathing and if they stop breathing, they will go into cardiac arrest, when the heart stops beating and the dog dies.

However, after breathing stops, and before cardiac arrest, the heart can continue to beat for several minutes and this is when performing cardiopulmonary resuscitation (CPR) or artificial respiration can save your dog's life.

Step 1: place your dog on his or her side on a flat surface.

Step 2: check to make sure that your dog has actually stopped breathing by watching for the rise and fall of their chest and feel for their breath on your hand. Check the color of your dog's gums, because lack of oxygen will make them turn blue.

Step 3: check that the dog's airway is clear and there is nothing stuck in their mouth or throat by extending the head and neck and opening your dog's mouth.

If there is an object blocking their throat, pull the tongue outward and use your fingers or pliers to get a firm grip on the object so that you can pull it free from the dog's throat. If you cannot reach the object that appears to be blocking the dog's airway passage, you will have to use the Heimlich Manoeuver to try and dislodge it (see below).

Step 4: so long as the dog's airway is not blocked, you can lift their chin to straighten out the neck and begin rescue breathing.

Step 5: hold the dog's muzzle and close their mouth, put your mouth over the dog's nose and blow gently – just enough to cause the dog's chest to rise.

Step 6: wait long enough for the air you just breathed into the dog's lungs to leave before giving another breath.

Step 7: continue giving one gentle breath every 3 seconds as long as the heart is still beating and until your dog starts to breathe on their own.

Canine Heimlich Manoeuvre

If breath won't go in, the airway may be blocked. In this case, you will need to turn your dog upside down, with his or her back held against your chest.

Wrap your arms around the dog and clasp your hands together just below the dog's rib cage (since the dog is being held upside down, this will be actually above the rib cage, in the abdomen).

Using both arms, give five sharp thrusts to the abdomen, and then check the dog's mouth or airway for the object. If the object is visible, remove it, and give two more rescue breaths.

CPR Step by Step

If your Cavapoo's heart has stopped beating, then CPR must be started immediately and ideal would be to have one person performing the artificial respiration, while the other performs the CPR.

Step 1: put your dog on his or her side on a flat surface.

Step 2: feel for your dog's pulse or heartbeat by placing one hand over his or her left side, just behind the front leg.

Step 3: place the palm of your hand on your dog's rib cage over his or her heart, with your other hand on top of the first (for puppies, put just your thumb on one side of the chest and the rest of your fingers on the other side).

Step 4: press down and release, compressing the dog's chest approximately one inch (2-3 centimetres) and squeeze and release 80 to 100 times every minute.

While it's always the hope that you may never need to, if your dog is not breathing and there is no pulse, knowing what steps to take in an emergency (which includes how to do the doggy Heimlich Manoeuvre or apply compressions), could literally save the life of your own dog or maybe even someone else's.

In a Nutshell

While generally crossbred dogs are healthier, and your dog may never suffer from any of the diseases known to occur in either breed parent, you will want to know what *may* afflict your dog because being aware of the signs can help them live a longer life. As well, familiarizing yourself with emergency CPR procedures in the following American Red Cross chart could help you save your dog's life.

It is also prudent to take the time to choose a veterinarian that can provide yearly check-ups, have your dog spayed or neutered in a timely fashion and educate yourself about required vaccinations.

Taking the steps outlined in this Chapter will help ensure that your Cavapoo will always have the best opportunity to be healthy and happy throughout your lifelong journey.

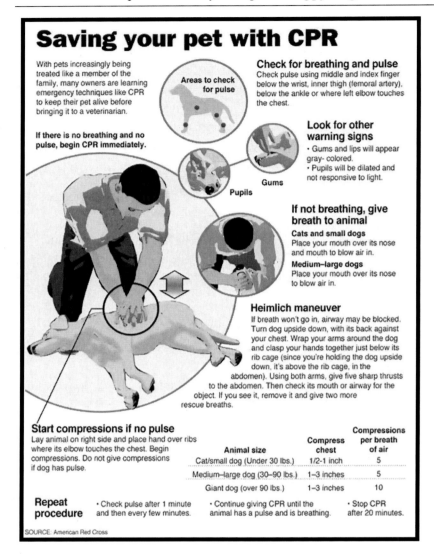

Saving your pet with CPR

With pets increasingly being treated like a member of the family, many owners are learning emergency techniques like CPR to keep their pet alive before bringing it to a veterinarian.

If there is no breathing and no pulse, begin CPR immediately.

Areas to check for pulse

Check for breathing and pulse
Check pulse using middle and index finger below the wrist, inner thigh (femoral artery), below the ankle or where left elbow touches the chest.

Look for other warning signs
· Gums and lips will appear gray- colored.
· Pupils will be dilated and not responsive to light.

Gums
Pupils

If not breathing, give breath to animal
Cats and small dogs
Place your mouth over its nose and mouth to blow air in.
Medium–large dogs
Place your mouth over its nose to blow air in.

Heimlich maneuver
If breath won't go in, airway may be blocked. Turn dog upside down, with its back against your chest. Wrap your arms around the dog and clasp your hands together just below its rib cage (since you're holding the dog upside down, it's above the rib cage, in the abdomen). Using both arms, give five sharp thrusts to the abdomen. Then check its mouth or airway for the object. If you see it, remove it and give two more rescue breaths.

Start compressions if no pulse
Lay animal on right side and place hand over ribs where its elbow touches the chest. Begin compressions. Do not give compressions if dog has pulse.

Animal size	Compress chest	Compressions per breath of air
Cat/small dog (Under 30 lbs.)	1/2-1 inch	5
Medium–large dog (30–90 lbs.)	1–3 inches	5
Giant dog (over 90 lbs.)	1–3 inches	10

Repeat procedure
· Check pulse after 1 minute and then every few minutes.
· Continue giving CPR until the animal has a pulse and is breathing.
· Stop CPR after 20 minutes.

SOURCE: American Red Cross

Chapter 5: Let Your Dog BE a Happy Dog

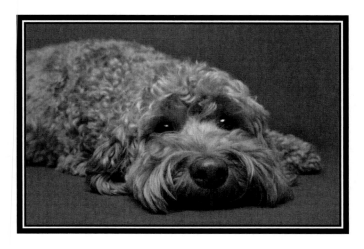

"Don't make the mistake of treating your dogs
like humans, or they'll treat you like dogs."
— Martha Scott

This chapter is written to alert you to the fact that far too many of us humans have the tendency to treat our dogs more like human fur children than dogs.

You need to understand that not allowing your Cavapoo to be *"dog-like"* is very important when we're talking about THEIR happiness, because treating a dog like a human can ultimately result in <u>you</u> creating any number of behavioral issues.

<u>Your Cavapoo is Not a Child</u>

While this might sound like a strange Chapter title, there is no doubt that many humans simply don't allow their dogs to actually BE dogs, because they are too busy confusing their dog by attributing human emotions to them, and treating them like children.

Yes, some dogs, such as the Cavapoo, may need to wear clothing to keep warm and dry, and depending on where they live and whether their coat is regularly clipped short, their guardian may need to provide them with protection from the cold and rain during the winter months. However, if the only reason you are dressing up your dog is because it makes you laugh, or appeals to a maternal instinct, this is not a healthy relationship.

The Cavapoo coat is often regularly clipped short (Puppy Clip) approximately every six weeks, because this is much easier to maintain than a Cavapoo in full, long coat that may easily mat. This means they may need to wear a sweater or coat on colder days and certainly a raincoat if you live in a rainy climate.

Also keep in mind that if you live in a warm climate, you may want to provide them with a cooling vest during warmer summer months when they are walking outside in the sunshine..

When your intelligent Cavapoo is a full-grown adult (approximately two years of age), you will definitely want to begin more complicated or advanced training sessions. They will enjoy it when you have the desire and patience, and they have the willingness.

If you and your Cavapoo are really enjoying learning new tricks together, you might want to advance to teaching them the hand signals for *"commando crawl"*, how to *"speak"* or to *"jump through the human hoop"*, and you might want to also consider getting them involved in a fun canine sport, like Agility.

You may be surprised at how capable this designer companion dog may be at learning many tricks and routines, which are fun to teach and will exercise both mind and body. The more control you have over your dog, the easier it will be to teach them a fun canine sport. Remember, half of this dog's DNA is Poodle, which means he or she will usually be an intelligent, quick to learn and agile performer that can really excel in the trick training department.

The only restriction to how far you can go with training your adult Cavapoo will be your imagination and their personal energy level, ability or desire to perform.

Every dog has a uniquely wonderful set of gifts to share with their human counterparts, if only us humans would listen. They *"tell"* us when they are unhappy, frightened, bored, nervous, and when they are under-exercised, yet often we do not pay attention, or we just think they are being badly behaved.

Many humans today are deciding to have dogs instead of children and then attempting to manipulate their dogs into being small (or large) furry children. This is having a seriously detrimental effect upon the health, happiness and behavior of our canine companions.

Single, lonely people often have dogs, which is just fine, so long as the human side of the equation doesn't expect their canine counterpart to fulfill what humans require on an emotional level, because this is very confusing to a dog who needs their human to lead them.

In order to be the best guardians for our dogs, we humans must have a better understanding of what our dogs need from us, rather than what we need from them, so that they can live in safety, harmony and security within our human environment.

Sadly, many of us humans are not well equipped to give our dogs what they really need and that is why there are so many homeless, abandoned and frustrated dogs and so many overflowing rescue facilities.

As a professional dog whisperer who is challenged with the task of finding amicable solutions for canine/human relationships that have gone off the rails, I can tell you with certainty that once humans understand what needs to be changed and actually take the steps to do the work required, almost every stressful canine/human relationship can be turned into a happy one.

The sad part is that many humans are simply not willing or able to really understand the breed they are choosing, or willing or able to do the consistent work and devote the time necessary to ensuring that their chosen dog's needs are met.

Almost ALL canine problems, both mentally and physically, are a direct result of ignorance, time restraints or unwillingness on the part of the human guardian to choose the right dog and then learn what their dog truly needs.

First and foremost, our dogs need to be respected for their unique canine qualities.

For millennia, dog has been considered *"Man's best friend"*. In today's society, when we want to do the best for our canine companions and create a harmonious relationship, we humans need to spend more time receiving the proper training WE need, so that we can learn how we humans can be dog's best friend.

Any dog can be your *"best friend"* providing that YOU educate yourself and put in the work. This is a universal truth that applies to any canine breed, including the smaller-sized Cavapoo.

If you are considering this affectionate and playful small dog for your family, be certain that you can involve them in a wide variety of routines and tasks that will engage both their body and their mind, because doing so will ensure that you are raising a happy dog that never has to suffer from behavioral issues or poor health.

In a Nutshell

It's important to understand that you actually need to let your dog BE a dog if you want to raise a happy and healthy companion.

While being overly protective, carrying this small dog everywhere and treating them like a fur covered child may be something YOU need, it's not what THEY need, and can create much confusion that often will lead to behavioral issues sooner or later in life.

Chapter 6: Every Happy Cavapoo Wants Exercise

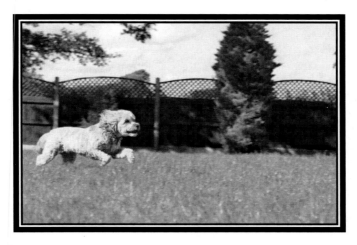

"The dog lives for the day,
the hour, even the moment."
— Robert Scott

This breed will usually require a moderate daily physical exercise regimen, that also includes going out for 2-3 on-leash walks, walking properly at your side every day, because this will result in a strong bond of trust and respect between you and your dog that translates to both a healthy body and a healthy mind.

If you cannot commit to the time required to ensure your dog receives regular exercise each day, that engages both mind and body, this will soon be a very unhealthy, overweight, unhappy dog that could develop multiple health and behavior issues.

Minimum Daily Exercise Requirements

You will need to get your dog outside every day for a minimum of two or three 20-40 minute, on-leash, disciplined walks where they are walking at your side without pulling, and paying close attention to your commands. Of course, if you like a longer walk, so will your Cavapoo.

Once properly leash trained and heeding basic commands, the Cavapoo will also enjoy the reward of some off-leash freedom at a securely fenced local dog park where they can run, socialize, play with other similar-sized dogs or chase a ball or small Frisbee. Also, many of these friendly little dogs like to snatch a ball away from another dog to get the other dog to chase them, so get into the habit of a daily visit to your local dog park.

Keep in mind that this small companion will usually be curious, fun loving and playful, and because they are a smaller, sturdy size, they are easy to travel with and great with children of all ages, which makes them popular family dogs.

TIP: get this small dog used to quietly travelling inside a handy *"Sherpa"* bag when he or she is a small puppy. When you take the time to do this, this little companion will easily travel anywhere with you, even on the local bus service or as carry-on luggage on a plane.

Ideal Daily Exercise Requirements

A fully-grown Cavapoo can be a curious, energetic and playful dog with plenty of stamina or (depending on you) more of a lazy couch potato. However, both will need mental and physical stimulation from disciplined walks and daily exercise, and that may include trick training or canine sports in order to maintain a happy disposition and a healthy weight.

Keep in mind that, depending on the particular dog and how you raise them, they will generally be more or less energetic. This means that if you are more energetic and enjoy getting out for plenty of walks or play at the local park, your dog will grow up to enjoy these activities too. It's a simple formula: you are more energetic, your dog is more energetic and both of you will be healthier and happier.

For instance, I've had Cavapoo clients whose dogs were calm, quiet, snoozy (and overweight), and others whose dogs loved getting outside and participating in energetic pursuits, so long as the weather was not too hot or cold. In other words, if you're active, your dog most likely will be, too.

A healthy Cavapoo will need to burn off their daily pent up energy by going for at least two to three good walks of 30 or 40 minutes or longer each beside their human companions every day, plus have an opportunity to run free chasing a ball or Frisbee, or playing and socializing amidst a pack of dogs, in a secure off-leash area.

In order for this social and affectionate little dog to be happy and well balanced, they will want to be involved in the family's activities and taken everywhere with you, which also helps to socialize, exercise their brains and prevent them from becoming bored, lazy or overweight.

Leaving a loving, affectionate dog alone for many hours every day that has been bred to be a canine companion, will be torture for them that could result in this dog becoming depressed, or making his or her own entertainment by becoming destructive and/or noisy by barking or crying.

The Cavapoo, in order to maintain a healthy weight, will require daily moderate exercising. Keep in mind that if this dog is permitted to become lazy and inactive, they will quickly gain weight, which can contribute to future health issues. There are far too many fat Cavapoos in the world today.

A very good way to give this dog the amount of physical and mental exercise they really need is to teach them to perform simple tricks, or train them to run an Agility course. When well socialized, this affectionate and sweet-natured dog could also be a wonderful therapy dog for those living in care facilities that are missing having a dog as part of their life. I've taken my Boris into many care facilities and those who are otherwise having a boring day immediately light up and are so happy to see him. Also, the Cavapoo can lower blood pressure without medication, because they have such wonderfully silky and soft fur that is a pleasure to stroke.

Ideal Living Conditions for a Happy Cavapoo

This friendly and affectionate companion is the perfect candidate for sharing life in a smaller, condominium or apartment-sized space, so long as you make the effort to ensure that they get outside for their disciplined, on-leash walks, play and socializing every day.

There is no doubt that the sweet natured Cavapoo, although lower to the ground than many other breeds, is a stout and sturdy companion with a loving personality and will enjoy plenty of attention and being close to you throughout whatever you're doing in your day.

Also, keep in mind that while this amusing little character can sometimes be stubborn (especially if they think the leadership role has defaulted to them), the personality of every Cavapoo will be different and they will develop traits and quirks that are unique to each dog.

While how each dog will develop will depend upon the temperament of the parents, the home where they are raised and how they are trained and socialized, the Cavapoo is generally a sensitive, happy, intelligent, eager to please student that may enjoy, for instance, running an Agility course or Advanced Obedience. This dog will respond well to fair, fun and consistent training programs involving treat-based reinforcement.

Many guardians of this breed will agree that their versatile little companions will faithfully follow them from room to room, as if attached by an invisible umbilical cord, because they just don't like to be left alone.

Properly socializing a Cavapoo early on, during the first three months of his or her life, will greatly influence the dog's temperament, personality and behavior as he or she matures into adulthood. Continuing to shape the personality of the dog through adolescence and on into adulthood with proper socializing, training, exercise, rules and boundaries, will ensure a well-mannered dog.

You'll also find that it's very difficult to get upset with a dog that only wants to spend all of their time in your company, especially when they're gazing lovingly at you with those big pleading eyes and a sweet, soulful expression that could turn even the stoniest of hearts to mush.

If you are unable to commit to providing the proper routine for this dog on a daily basis, that includes on-going socialization, training, and spending the majority of his or her time in your company, this loving companion will very likely first become unhealthily overweight, and second, may easily become nervous, anxious and suffer from separation anxiety. A dog that is suffering in this way, unlike some other behavioral issues, can take much patience and a very long time to turn around.

An under-exercised dog will become fat, bored and unhappy, which can then cause them to develop behavioral problems that could include acting out in destructive ways by chewing *"off limits"* items in the home, digging holes in the garden, escaping the back yard and ultimately suffering from anxiety and stress that can prematurely shorten their life.

In order to raise a happy Cavapoo that will be a contented member of your family, it will be essential that you provide him or her with moderate daily disciplined walks and the opportunity for play time in the local park or competing in a fun canine sport (where they get to use their mind), in order to maintain a happy disposition and a healthy weight.

The best you can do for this sweet, fun-loving companion is to properly train, socialize and exercise them every day beginning from the time when you first bring them home from the breeders.

Above all else, never forget that all dogs (no matter their size) are pack animals, which means that it is not normal for them to spend long periods of time by themselves. This is even more important with a dog that has been bred to be a family companion, such as the Cavapoo. Always remember that when you adopt a dog into your family you become their pack and you cannot simply abandon them when it's convenient for you to do so.

In other words, if you're planning to leave your companion alone for many hours every day, while you're at work or out for an evening at the pub with friends, don't get a Cavapoo (or ANY dog for that matter); if you do, you will undoubtedly be contributing to your fur friend developing a depressed and unhappy state of mind, and where the Cavapoo is concerned, most likely depression, nervousness and the stress of separation anxiety.

As well, when a bored Cavapoo has to find ways to entertain his or herself, you will also be opening the door to your loyal and affectionate dog developing unwanted behaviors. These behaviors can include becoming destructive, barking or whining and crying until they become hoarse, or attempting to escape so they can wander the neighborhood in search of their humans, that could lure them far away from home.

In a Nutshell

The bottom line here is that the Cavapoo is an affectionate, loving, and always sweet, and playful small companion that requires several walks every day, plus the opportunity for play, learning new tricks and routines or canine sports, and time to socialize with other dogs and people.

This Chapter also outlines several different canine sports that an energetic Cavapoo may excel at, such as Agility, or Trick Training. Truly consider involving this dog in a sport, because this is a great way to provide them with the exercise they need in a disciplined way that will engage their mind and help to ensure that your dog is a healthy and happy family member, while also teaching them that you are their leader.

Take Away Tip: *while this dog usually needs a moderate amount of daily exercise, they also need maximum time in your company and will excel when you provide them with a daily routine that takes into consideration what is appropriate for their best physical and mental health.*

Chapter 7: Feeding the Happy Cavapoo

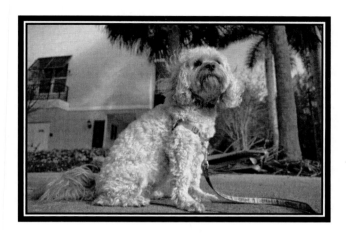

"I feel sorry for people who don't have dogs.
I hear they have to pick up food they drop on the floor."
— Unknown

It's not rocket science to grasp the concept that a properly fed Cavapoo means a healthy, happy and longer-lived companion, so make sure that you spend an appropriate amount of time to research high-quality food and treats that will be the best for your happy Cavapoo.

We are what we eat, and the same is absolutely true for our canine companions. Often this breed can develop picky eating habits, so make sure that you don't get into the habit of *"doctoring"* their food bowl with your human food. If you do, your dog may soon refuse to eat their doggy dinner. Don't worry, though, because even a picky eater will not starve him or herself, and if they refuse their expensive dog dinner tonight, so long as you don't cave, they WILL be hungry tomorrow.

First, remember that our canine friends are carnivores, which means that they derive their energy and nutrient requirements and maintain their health by consuming a diet consisting mainly or exclusively of the flesh of animal tissues. In other words, your dog is a meat eater.

When choosing an appropriate diet for your Cavapoo, considering the physiology of the canine's teeth, jaws and digestive tract will give you a better understanding of what food they should be eating.

Teeth, Jaws, and Digestive Tract

Teeth: canine teeth are all pointed because they are designed to rip, shred and tear into animal meat and bone.

Jaws: every canine is born equipped with powerful jaws and neck muscles for the specific purpose of being able to pull down and tear apart their hunted prey.

The jaw of every canine opens widely to hold large pieces of meat and bone, while the actual mechanics of the canine jaw permits only vertical (up and down) movement that is designed for crushing.

Digestive Tract: the canine digestive tract is short, simple and designed to move their natural choice of food (hide, meat and bone) quickly through their systems.

We humans need vegetables and plant matter in our diet and have the flat molars to effectively crush and chew them. While we often believe our dogs require the same, when choosing an appropriate food source for your Cavapoo, you need to consider that vegetables and plant matter require more time to break down in the gastrointestinal tract. This in turn, requires a more complex digestive system that the canine body simply does not have.

The canine digestive system is unable to break down vegetable matter, which is why whole vegetables look pretty much the same going into your dog, as they do coming out the other end.

Consider how much healthier and long-lived your beloved Cavapoo can be if, instead of largely ignoring nature's design for our canine companions, we chose to feed them whole, unprocessed, species-appropriate food.

Whatever you decide to feed your dog, keep in mind that, just as too much wheat or other grains and fillers in our human diet are having detrimental effects on our human health, the same can be very true for our dogs.

Read the labels so that you can be certain to avoid foods that contain fillers or high amounts of grains, because these are inappropriate for a healthy canine diet.

Control of Your Happy Cavapoo's Food

The Cavapoo will usually have a moderately healthy appetite, although they can get bored with eating the same food every day, so mix it up a little. For instance, my dog, Boris, usually has little interest in food during the morning, but is ready for his dental treat at high noon. His internal clock is spot on and if I'm not paying attention to the time, he just calmly sits there staring at me until I get it.

It's important that your Cavapoo understands that YOU are in control of their food source. Once they understand this, they will also figure out that there will be windows of opportunity for receiving and eating their food, and this routine will help to develop healthy eating habits.

Many people use a scoop or measuring cup to put dry food into their dog's bowl. This is a mistake, because it's very important to mix your dog's food with your hands, so that your scent is all over the food, before you give it to them to eat. This sends a "message" to your dog that you are their pack leader, because it mimics what would happen if you were the alpha dog out hunting for your food in the wild.

For instance, while a pack of wild dogs hunting for food all work hard to capture their prey, the alpha pack leader always gets to eat first while all the other dogs must wait until the leader of the pack eats their fill, before they can rush in to eat what is left over.

Therefore, when you are mixing your domesticated dog's dinner with your hands, you are sending them the subtle message that you are the pack leader, you've already eaten your fill and you are now allowing them to eat what was left over.

Feeding Puppies

A general rule of thumb for growing Cavapoo puppies is to feed daily amounts of between 2 and 3% of what the puppy's adult weight is projected to be or 10% of the puppy's current body weight. You will want to keep in mind that while all puppies require extra protein during the first two years of their life to help them develop into healthy adult dogs, this is especially important with higher energy puppies.

You will also want to keep a close eye to make sure that this tiny puppy is eating and drinking enough throughout the day, so set regular feeding times each day.

There are now many foods on the market that are formulated for all stages of a dog's life (including the puppy stage). Whether you choose one of these foods or a food specially formulated for puppies, they will need to be fed smaller meals more frequently throughout the day (between 3 and 5 times), until they are at least one year of age.

Feeding Adults

Choose foods that list high-quality meat protein as the main ingredient and, depending on your dog's particular energy level, feed between 2 and 3% of their body weight every day. While some dogs prefer one meal a day, most will appreciate morning food (after a walk) and evening food (after a walk).

Be careful not to get caught up in "convenience" when you are out grocery shopping for yourself, and decide to buy your Cavapoo's food at the same place, because most grocery stores tend to carry inferior brands of dog food.

Instead, make the time to visit your local pet store, talk with educated representatives, avoid grains, and choose quality sources of meat protein for healthy puppies and dogs, including beef, buffalo, chicken, duck, fish, hare, lamb, ostrich, pork, rabbit, turkey, venison, or any other source of wild meaty protein.

Treats

There are endless choices of dog treats lining the shelves of every feed store, pet store, and grocery store, and it will be an overwhelming task to choose wisely, unless you keep one simple rule in mind, and choose treats that contain only one ingredient or very few ingredients.

Whatever reason you choose to give treats to your Cavapoo, keep in mind that if we treat our dogs too often throughout the day, they can become overweight, and we may create a picky eater who will no longer want to eat their regular meals. Think about it – if you got to eat only your favourite tasty treats throughout the day, would you be excited about consuming a less flavourful meal come dinner time?

As well, researchers in Sweden have discovered that dogs were happier when they had to <u>earn</u> their treats as a reward for completing a task, rather than just being given a treat for looking cute, because just like us humans who get that happy "eureka" moment when we finally solve a problem, the same is true for our canine counterparts. The eager to learn Cavapoo is the perfect dog for positive training methods that involve treat reinforcement.

Dangerous Treats

Always carefully read labels and take note of where treats are manufactured, because not all countries have the most stringent manufacturing protocols, and honestly there are many treats that you absolutely should NOT be feeding your dog, including:

Rawhide, which is soaked in an ash/lye solution to remove every particle of meat, fat and hair and then further soaked in bleach to remove remaining traces of the ash/lye solution. Now that the product is no longer food, it no longer has to comply with food regulations.

The wet rawhide is shaped into chews, and once dry it shrinks to approximately 25% of its original size before arsenic-based products are used as preservatives, and antibiotics and insecticides are added to kill bacteria.

While rawhide chews are tough and long lasting, when a dog chews a rawhide treat, they ingest many harsh chemicals. Also, when your dog swallows a piece of rawhide, that piece can swell up to four times its size inside your dog's stomach, which can cause anything from mild to severe gastric blockages that could become life threatening and require surgery. As much as it might be convenient for you to be able to give your dog or puppy a treat that will occupy them for a considerable time, if it's rawhide, just say "No".

Pig's Ears are very attractive to most dogs that will eagerly devour them, and they're "natural" because they're ears, so what could be wrong? Actually, these are thin, crispy and very high in fat, which can cause stomach upsets, vomiting and diarrhoea. In addition, pieces can break off and become stuck in a dog's throat.

Also, pig ears are often processed and preserved with unhealthy chemicals that discerning dog guardians will not want to feed their dogs. Just say "No".

Hoof Treats are actual cow, horse and pig hooves that humans believe are healthy, *"natural"* treat choices for their dogs when the truth is that after processing with harsh chemicals, preservatives and antibiotics, they retain little, if any, of their *"natural"* qualities.

Also, hooves are very hard and can cause the chipping or breaking of your dog's teeth as well as perforation or blockages in your dog's intestines. Just say "No".

Healthy Treats

There are so many healthy treat choices available, which means that there is no excuse for feeding your Cavapoo unhealthy, nutrient-deficient treats that could harm them. Read the labels to make sure the treats you are choosing are appropriately sized for your dog and are of the highest quality. Examples of healthy treats include:

Hard Treats: come in many varieties of shapes, sizes and flavors and will help to keep your dog's teeth cleaner.

Soft Treats: are also available in endless varieties and flavors, suitable for all the different needs of our furry friends and are often smaller in size and used for training purposes.

Dental Treats or Chews: are designed with the specific purpose of helping your dog to maintain healthy teeth and gums by exercising the jaw and massaging gums, while removing plaque build-up near the gum line. Providing a daily dental chew will be especially important with a dog like the Cavapoo, that has a smaller jaw and is more likely to develop dental issues.

Freeze-Dried and Jerky Treats: offer a tasty morsel most dogs find irresistible as they are usually made of simple, meaty ingredients, such as liver, poultry and seafood. Be careful when choosing jerky treats, as they are often processed with too much salt.

Human Food Treats: be very careful when feeding human foods to dogs as treats, because many of our foods contain unhealthy additives, such as salt, sugar and other ingredients that could be toxic and harmful.

Also, educate yourself about the common human foods that are actually poisonous to our canine friends, such as grapes, raisins, onions and chocolate, to name a few.

Generally, the treats you feed your dog should not make up more than approximately 10% of their daily food intake, so make sure the treats you choose are high quality, with single or few ingredients so that you can help to keep your Cavapoo both happy and healthy.

The Right Food for Your Happy Cavapoo

"Dog Food" has significantly changed since 1785, when the English Sportman's Dictionary described the best diet for a dog's health in an article entitled *"Dog"*. This article indicated that the best food for a dog was something called *"Greaves"*, described as "*the sediment of melted tallow made into cakes for dogs' food*".

From these meager beginnings, commercially manufactured dog food has become a massively lucrative industry that has only fairly recently evolved beyond feeding our dogs the dregs of human leftovers, because it was cheap and convenient for us.

Even today, the majority of dog food choices often have far more to do with being convenient for humans to store and serve, than it does with being a diet truly designed to be a nutritionally balanced, healthy food choice for our canine companions.

Educating yourself by talking to experts and reading everything you can find on the subject, plus taking into consideration several relevant factors, will help to answer the dog food question for you and your dog.

For instance, where you live may dictate what sorts of foods you have access to, while other factors to consider will include the particular requirements of your dog, such as their age, energy and activity levels.

Our dogs are also suffering from many of the same life-threatening diseases that are commonly found in our human society (heart disease, cancer, diabetes, obesity). These diseases all have a direct correlation with over-feeding and/or eating genetically altered foods that are no longer pure, in favor of a convenient, processed and packaged diet that is quick and easy for us to serve.

The Raw Diet: raw feeding advocates believe that the ideal diet for their dog is one which would be very similar to what a dog living in the wild would have access to while hunting or foraging.

These canine guardians are often opposed to feeding their dog any sort of commercially manufactured pet foods, because they consider them to be poor substitutes, and for the most part, I would agree.

For instance, many guardians of high energy, working breed dogs will agree that their dogs thrive on a raw or BARF (Biologically Appropriate Raw Food) diet and strongly believe that the potential benefits of feeding a raw dog food diet are many, whether your dog is earning a daily working wage or simply being your loyal companion, including:

- Healthy, shiny coats

- Decreased shedding

- Fewer allergy problems

- Healthier skin

- Cleaner teeth

- Fresher breath

- Increased energy levels

- Improved digestion

- Smaller stools

- Strengthened immune system

- Increased mobility in arthritic pets

- Increase or improvement in overall health

A raw diet is a direct evolution of what dogs ate before they became our domesticated pets and we turned toward commercially prepared, easy-to-serve dry dog food that required no special storage or preparation.

The Dehydrated Diet: is available in both raw and cooked meat forms, which are usually air dried to reduce moisture and inhibit bacterial growth. While the appearance of dehydrated dog food is very similar to dry kibble, the typical feeding methods include adding warm water before serving, which makes this type of diet both healthy for our dogs and convenient for us to serve.

Dehydrated recipes are made from minimally processed fresh, whole foods to create a healthy and nutritionally balanced meal that retains more of the overall nutritional value, and will meet or exceed the dietary requirements of a healthy canine.

A dehydrated diet is a convenient way to feed your dog a nutritious diet, because all you have to do is add warm water and wait five minutes while the food re-hydrates so your dog can enjoy a warm meal.

The Kibble Diet: there is no mistaking that the convenience and relative economy of dry dog food kibble, which had its beginnings in the 1940's, continues to be the most popular pet food choice for many dog-friendly humans. Thankfully, there are now many high-quality kibble foods available.

The Right Bowl for the Cavapoo: there are many different types and categories of dog bowls, including Automatic Watering, Elevated, Ceramic, Stoneware, No Skid, No Tip, Slow Feeder, Stainless, Wooden and Travel Bowls. Always purchase bowls that are appropriately sized for your particular dog, and consider an elevated dining table so that their head is up from the floor when eating and drinking.

In a Nutshell

While food and treat choices for your favorite furry Cavapoo can be overwhelming, a basic understanding of canine physiology and making wise decisions concerning all the many different types of food and treats available, will help you to add many healthy and happy years to your dog's life.

You are the sole protector of your canine companion, and I cannot stress strongly enough the importance of a well thought out choice when deciding what brand and type of food and treats you will feed your loyal canine companion.

Appropriate food/treat choices and being careful to not overfeed, may not only increase the length of your dog's life by avoiding unwanted health conditions, such as obesity, high blood pressure or bladder stones, good food choices will also provide your dog with optimal health so they can feel good and live a happy life!

Chapter 8: Care of the Happy Cavapoo

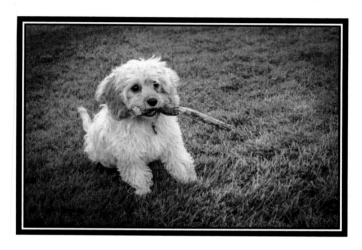

*"When you adopt a dog, you have a lot of
very good days, and one very bad day."*
— W. Bruce Cameron

Imagine you're travelling by car on a daily basis without being
protected by a seatbelt or an airbag. How safe would you feel?
Unfortunately, this is the reality for far too many of our furry friends,
because their guardians have neglected their safety responsibilities.

Now, imagine going for months without washing your hair, cutting your
nails or brushing your teeth. Again, that is the reality for many dogs,
because their owners have not been advised with respect to the
importance of good grooming. How happy and well-behaved do you
think such an ill cared for dog would be?

The following few paragraphs outline safe travelling, licensing,
insurance and grooming requirements, all of which can help to ensure
that your Cavapoo is safe, legal and better cared for at the vet's office.

Keep in mind that if your dog is safely secured when travelling, they
might not be dead or seriously injured should you be involved in a

vehicle accident. We humans wear seatbelts to be safe – what about safety for our best fur friends?

Further, if your dog is properly licensed, they will be returned to you should they go missing, and this is a much happier dog than one spending who knows how long behind bars at a rescue or SPCA.

As well, if you have pet health insurance, chances are that your dog will be better cared for at the vet's office, which means a healthier and happier companion.

Tips for Keeping Your Dog Safe

Not So Safe Harness Restraints: is your canine companion safe when buckled into a safety harness for travel in vehicles? Be aware that many of the dog harnesses in the marketplace have a 100% failure rate.

If you cannot find a safety harness that is actually been strength tested and crash tested (i.e. optimal choice), the safest travel arrangement for any dog is to secure them inside a kennel, that is bolted to the floor or secured with the vehicles seatbelt. Remember that a dog travelling in the front passenger seat, even one secured with a proper safety harness, may still sustain injuries (and even death) if the 100 mph force of the airbag strikes them.

Kennels: a dog kennel or crate will easily fit (sideways) on the back seat of most vehicles and can be secured with the vehicle's restraint system. A Cavapoo riding inside a kennel that is secure inside your vehicle will have the best protection in the case of a rollover accident, plus you will avoid the fines some locations are now levying for allowing a dog to roam freely inside a moving vehicle.

Air Travel: the Cavapoo puppy will be small enough to fit into a soft Sherpa bag for travel inside an airplane cabin (as carry-on baggage), and most, depending on their size, may remain small enough to travel as carry-on luggage inside the airplane cabin when they are fully grown. Any dogs that are too large to fit comfortably inside a Sherpa travel bag will need to be transported inside a heated cargo hold.

Licensing: when you purchase your dog a yearly license or identifying tag, they will be legal, and should they become lost when wearing a license, there is a much higher possibility that your dog will be returned to you, instead of spending their last few days behind bars at the local SPCA or rescue facility.

Pet Health Insurance: purchasing health insurance for your dog means that they will usually live a longer, healthier and happier life, because they will receive better care throughout their lifetime.

Be aware that you need to begin insurance when your dog is a young puppy, because waiting until they are older will mean that your monthly premiums are considerably higher.

Grooming Your Dog

Regular grooming is important for a happy and healthy Cavapoo, because it keeps them clean, their skin moisturized and bug free, plus grooming time can alert you to any problems before they become more serious. This dog's hair may be constantly growing and may not shed, which means that you will need to have him or her professionally groomed approximately every six weeks. It will also be a good idea to commit to at least a weekly brushing to remove debris and any matted hair.

Depending upon whether you decide to fully groom your dog yourself, or will take him or her to the local doggy spa, you will require minimal or much more equipment to keep the coat of your happy Cavapoo looking his or her best. If you're just keeping on top of weekly brushing, all you will need is a soft bristle brush, and perhaps a flea comb (just in case). If you're planning to do all your dog's grooming yourself, see *"Grooming Equipment You Will Need"* on the next page.

Also, you will want to get your dog used to their grooming routine early on, because otherwise, every time your dog needs to be bathed or brushed will end up being a traumatic experience for both dog and human that can last for many years. Start them off right so you can both enjoy grooming time.

For instance, I've been asked to groom dogs that have been kicked out of every grooming salon because their owners did not take the time to introduce the puppy to bath time, nail clipping and other necessary grooming procedures at a young age.

I can tell you from much personal experience that having to groom a writhing, screaming dog that is all teeth, because they are fighting the procedure, is hell on wheels, and the very worst case I ever encountered was with a dog weighing only 4 pounds (1.8 kg). Try going through this with a sturdy, unwilling Cavapoo, and you will very soon be wishing your companion were a chia pet.

Grooming Equipment You Will Need

A standard arsenal of equipment for the DIY groomer that will help you keep your Cavapoo looking their best will include the following:

Electric Clipper – you will need a professional grade, quiet, two-speed clipper with detachable blades that can be corded or cordless (Andis, Wahl), and at least one or two blades, depending on what length you wish your dog's coat to be. I use a size 4F blade for keeping my Boris in an easy to manage "puppy clip".

Bristle brush – is the ideal tool for removing debris minimal mats from the Cavapoo's coat, while at the same time distributing natural oils to keep the coat looking healthy and shiny.

Set of Scissors – you will need a sharp, professional set of scissors for trimming around the tail, face, legs, feet and other tighter areas.

Sturdy Metal Comb – get one that has rotating teeth as this pulls the hair much less.

Slicker Brush – this has rows of metal teeth placed closely together and is a great tool for smoothing the coat before clipping.

Nail clippers or scissors (and/or a slow speed pet Dremel™) – will be tools you need to use every couple of weeks or more, depending on how quickly your Cavapoo's nails grow and what types of surfaces they may be walking on. The pet Dremel is perfect for smoothing the sharp edges that nail clippers leave, and if you are vigilant with regular use of the Dremel, you may never have to clip.

Flea comb – hopefully you won't ever need one, however, as the name suggests, these combs are designed for the specific purpose of removing fleas from a dog's coat. Usually small in size for manoeuvring in tight spaces, they may be made of plastic or metal with the teeth of the comb placed very close together to trap hiding fleas.

Tick Twister – hopefully your dog won't ever get a tick, but if they do, this is a simple device for painlessly, easily and quickly removing ticks that have imbedded themselves in your dog's skin.

Grooming Products You Will Need

Products you will need to invest in when bathing your dog yourself will include shampoos, conditioners, creams, lotions, sprays and powders.

Shampoos: NEVER make the mistake of using human shampoo or conditioner that has a pH balance of 5.5, for bathing your dog. Our canine companions have an almost neutral pH balance of 7.5, and any shampoo with a lower pH will be harmful to your dog, because it will strip the natural oils and be too harshly acidic for their coat and skin, which can create itchy skin problems and allow for a very unhappy dog.

Conditioners: taking the extra time to condition your Cavapoo's coat will not only make it look and feel better, it will also add additional benefits, including:

- Preventing the escape of natural oils and moisture
- Keeping the coat cleaner for a longer period of time
- Repairing a coat that has become dull, damaged or dry
- Restoring a soft, silky feel
- Helping the coat dry more quickly
- Protecting from the heat of the dryer and breakage of hair

The benefits of spending the extra two minutes to condition your dog's coat will be appreciated by both yourself and your dog that will have overall healthy, moisturized skin and a coat with a natural shine.

Oops, My Dog Has Fleas

You haven't been paying attention and now realize that your dog is suffering from an infestation of fleas. Now is the time to bathe them with shampoo containing pyrethrum (a botanical extract found in small, white daisies) or a shampoo containing citrus or tea tree oil.

Also, you can bathe and spray them with the non-toxic and highly effective CedarCide products, which can also be used to spray down their bedding and any carpets in the home, and will kill fleas (or other crawly creatures) on contact without harming anyone.

CedarCide is a company that makes 100% safe, organic products to control biting bugs on your furry friends without worrying about harmful chemicals that are not good for you, your children or your canine companions.

Simply spray it on and bugs of any sort that come into contact with the solution will be dead, while your dog's coat will be shiny and fresh smelling, like the inside of a cedar chest.

Nail Care

Many canine guardians neglect taking proper care of their dog's toenails, which can lead to many problems later in life, such as painful joints and difficulty walking, which will make for a very unhappy Cavapoo.

Purchase a good pair of medium-sized, scissor-type nail clippers with a safety stop and learn how to properly use them every two to three weeks. If you don't, your dog's nails will soon be too long and the vein inside the nail will also grow too long and you will be unable to keep them as short as they should be.

IMPORTANT: if your puppy has not had their "dew claws" removed (these are the claws that are on the side of the foot that never touch the ground), they still continue to grow. If you miss clipping these nails, they will soon grow into a circle that will be very difficult to clip and can even grow back into the leg causing great pain.

Styptic Powder: you will always want to avoid causing any pain when trimming your Cavapoo's toenails, because you don't want to destroy their trust in you regularly performing this necessary task.

However, accidents do happen, therefore if you clip too short, and accidentally cut into the vein in the toenail, know that you will cause your dog pain, and that the toenail will bleed. Therefore, it is always a good idea to keep some styptic powder (often called *"Kwik Stop")* in your grooming kit.

Dip a moistened finger into the powder and apply it with pressure to the end of the bleeding nail, because this is the quickest way to stop a nail from bleeding in just a few seconds.

Some dogs prefer having their nails trimmed with a rotary "Dremel" type of device that grinds down the excess nail. With this tool, it is easier to avoid cutting into the vein, and if you use this tool every week, you can trim shorter and will never have to actually clip the nails.

Keep in mind that if you decide to trim your dog's nails this way, you will have to purchase a *"doggy Dremel"* made especially for this purpose, because using your shop Dremel will harm your dog's nails as it is too high speed and will burn the nails.

Ear Care

Dogs can often suffer from painful ear infections, because the ears can easily retain moisture.

Paying attention and keeping your dog's ears clean and dry will prevent this type of unhappy pain and suffering. Make sure that you keep ear powders and cleaning solutions in your grooming kit, because with proper preventative care, your dog need never suffer from an ear infection.

Ear Powders: which can be purchased at any pet store, are designed to help keep your dog's ears dry while at the same time inhibiting the growth of bacteria that can lead to infections. Ear powders are also used when removing excess hair growth from inside a dog's ear canal, as the powder makes it easier to grip the hair.

Ear Cleaning Solutions: your local pet store will offer a wide variety of ear cleaning creams, drops, oils, rinses or wipes specially formulated for cleaning your Cavapoo's ears.

In addition, there are many home remedies that will just as efficiently clean your dog's ears without the high price tag, including Witch Hazel (a 50:50 solution of Organic Apple Cider Vinegar and Purified Water) or a 50:50 solution of Hydrogen Peroxide and Purified Water.

Teeth Care

Another greatly overlooked area in your happy Cavapoo's health is ensuring that their teeth are clean and properly looked after, so that they don't suffer from loose or broken teeth, and plaque build-up that leads to painful gum disease. You know how miserable a toothache can be – imagine your poor dog that cannot tell you how unhappy they are.

Proper teeth care that includes regular, daily brushing is VERY important with a smaller dog, like the Cavapoo, that has a smaller muzzle, because they are more prone to teeth problems and gum disease.

Many guardians use the excuse that *"my dog doesn't like it"* when they try to brush their dog's teeth, and overlook the fact that in order to keep their entire dog healthy, they <u>must</u> have healthy teeth and the only way to ensure this, is to commit to making the time to brush your dog's teeth every day.

Also remember that because the Cavapoo has a smaller jaw, they may have too many teeth packed in there, so ask your vet if any of them need to be removed around the same time as the puppy teeth are naturally falling out and the adult teeth are starting to come through (at around six months of age).

Canine Toothpastes: are flavoured with beef or chicken in an attempt to appeal to the dog's taste buds, while some contain baking soda, which is the same mild abrasive found in many human pastes, and are designed to gently scrub the teeth.

Other types of canine toothpastes are formulated with enzymes that are designed to work chemically by breaking down tartar or plaque in the dog's mouth. While these pastes don't need to be washed off your dog's teeth and are safe for them to swallow, whether or not they remain on the dog's teeth long enough to do any good might be debatable.

Just as effective for killing germs, whitening and cleaning your dog's teeth, and much less expensive than fancy pastes, is old-fashioned hydrogen peroxide; you can combine hydrogen peroxide (3% food grade), Aloe Vera juice (1:1) with a little bit of baking soda.

Paw Care

If your dog runs over sharp barnacles on the beach, jogs with you on hard road surfaces, or over other rough surfaces, this can cause cuts and scrapes and very rough surfaces on the paws. If you live in a hot climate, be aware that sidewalks, road surfaces and sandy beaches can get extremely hot for your Cavapoo's feet.

Paw Creams: depending upon activity levels and the types of surfaces our canine counterparts usually walk on, they may suffer from cracked or rough pads. You can restore resiliency and keep your dog's paws in healthy condition by regularly applying a cream or lotion to protect their paw pads. A good time to do this is just after you've clipped their nails.

In a Nutshell

Learning about simple steps that will keep your Cavapoo safe, and what's involved in keeping him or her properly groomed will go a long way toward helping them to live a long, happy and healthy life.

While for many people the concept of grooming your dog conjures up notions of brushes and bows, it is in fact a vital element to their overall health and wellbeing.

Regularly grooming your dog will help you detect any underlying diseases or conditions early and will allow your beloved fur friend to feel better and live longer and happier.

Chapter 9: Are YOU the Ideal Happy Cavapoo Guardian?

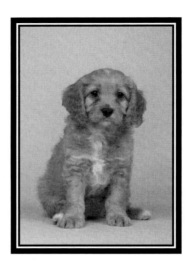

"A dog is the only thing on earth that
loves you more than he loves himself."
— Josh Billings

If you have not chosen wisely when sharing your life with a canine companion, you are setting yourself, your family, your friends and your neighbours up for many years of stress, guilt and unhappiness.

It is vitally important that you take a good hard look at your own energy level and lifestyle, ask yourself some serious questions that you honestly answer, and not scrimp on taking the time to do plenty of research about the breed of dog you may be considering.

Sharing your life with a canine friend should never be undertaken lightly, or on a whim or spur of the moment decision, or because you like the colour of a dog's coat or the sweet expression on their face.

Before you can learn how to become your dog's ideal guardian, you need to first have no doubt in your mind that you have the energy, commitment, time and skill level necessary to raise a happy dog. Once this is established in the affirmative, you then need to know how to choose the right breed of puppy or dog.

Choosing the right puppy for your family and your lifestyle is more important than you might imagine, and far too many people forget to consider how important is to choose a puppy or dog based on compatibility with their own energy and lifestyle.

For instance, many humans choose a puppy (or older dog) for all the wrong reasons, including because:

- they like what it looks like
- the breed may currently be popular
- the breed appeared on TV or in a movie they enjoyed
- their parents had the same kind of dog when they were a child
- a friend has the same breed
- they feel sorry for a homeless dog
- a friend or family member can no longer keep their dog
- the children are begging for a dog
- someone was selling puppies on a street corner

While some of these above reasons can be honourable, the most important reasons for choosing to share your life with a particular canine companion has not been properly considered.

In order to make an intelligent choice that will bring happiness to everyone, you need to take a serious look at your life as it is today and also how you envision it to be during the next ten to fifteen years, and then ask yourself several very important questions, including:

Activity – Do I lead a highly active, medium or low-intensity life? For instance, am I out jogging the streets every morning, hiking local mountains or riding my bicycle five miles to the local grocery store? Does my job keep me away from home, and does my leisure time activity keep me in front of the computer or on the couch watching movies?

Travel – Do I travel a lot for work or pleasure? If you do, perhaps you should choose a small dog that can travel with you in the plane cabin. Your loyal dog will be unhappy without you or you will have greatly increased expenses, because you will have to hire a dog sitter or leave them in a kennel.

Allergies – Do I prefer a very tidy house? Do I have allergies? Many breeds constantly shed their hair, which means that there are better choices for allergy sufferers and neat freaks.

Time – Does my family take up all my spare time and are my children old enough to handle a puppy? A dog is like a child that never grows up and in order for them to be happy and well-behaved family members, they require a lot of your daily time and attention.

Fitness – Am I physically fit and healthy enough to be out there walking a dog two to three times a day, every day, rain or shine, and much more during the puppy stage? Do I have the time to involve them in a canine sport or job?

Cost – Am I able to afford the extra food costs, trips to the grooming parlour, health insurance, licensing, appropriate clothing and the veterinarian expenses that are part of being a conscientious Cavapoo guardian?

Commitment – Is the decision to bring a puppy or dog into my life a family decision, or just because the children, who may quickly lose interest, have been begging for a dog?

Why? – What is the number one reason why I want a dog in my life?

Once you ask yourself these important questions and honestly answer them, you will have gained a much better understanding of whether or not you have what it takes to share your life with a dog, and perhaps the beginning insight of the type of puppy or dog that would be best suited for you and your family.

If you're too busy for a dog, or choose the wrong dog that is not compatible with you or your family's energy and lifestyle (or you don't really have the time, finances, patience, expertise and commitment necessary to properly socialize, train, exercise, feed, raise and care for a canine companion), you will inevitably end up with an unhappy dog, which will lead to behavioral issues, which then will lead to a stressed family, angry neighbors, and in a best case scenario, extra expenses to hire a professional to help you reverse unwanted behavioral problems.

Even worse, an incompatible choice can mean that you may end up contributing to the already overflowing crisis of yet another dog being abandoned at the local SPCA or kill shelter.

Once you have done all your homework, and absolutely determined that the friendly, little Cavapoo is the right dog for you (see next Section: The Ideal Guardian), rather than simply leaving it to chance, you need to choose the right puppy from the litter.

Generally speaking, when choosing a puppy out of a litter, look for one that is friendly and outgoing, rather than one who is overly aggressive or fearful.

Visit the breeder and take note of a puppy's social skills when they are still with their littermates, because this will help you to choose the right puppy for your family. Puppies who demonstrate good social skills with their littermates are much more likely to develop into easy-going, happy adults who play well with other dogs.

In a social setting where all the puppies can be observed together, there are several important observations you can make, including:

Play – Notice which puppies are comfortable both on top and on the bottom when play fighting and wresting with their littermates, and which puppies seem to only like being on top. Puppies who don't mind being on the bottom or who appear to be fine with either position will usually play well with other dogs when they become adults.

Sharing – Observe which puppies try to keep the toys away from the other puppies and which puppies share. Those who want to hoard the toys and keep all other puppies away may be more aggressive with other dogs over food or treats, or in play where toys are involved as they become older.

Company – Notice which puppies seem to like the company of the other pups and which ones seem to be loners. Puppies who like the company of their littermates are more likely to be interested in the company of other dogs as they mature than anti-social puppies.

Compassion – Observe the reaction of puppies that get yelped at when they bite or roughhouse with another puppy too hard. Puppies who ease up when another puppy yelps or cries are more likely to respond appropriately when they play too roughly as adults.

Sociability – Check to see if the puppy you are interested in is sociable with people, because if they will not come to you, or display fear of strangers, this may develop into a fear/aggression problem when they become adults.

Handling – Check if the puppy you are interested in is relaxed about being handled, because if they are not, they may become difficult or overly nervous around adults and children during daily interactions, during grooming or while visiting the veterinarian's office.

Is Your Happy Puppy Healthy?

While mental health is very important, you will also want to do all you can to determine if your chosen puppy is physically healthy.

First, ask to see veterinarian reports from the breeder to satisfy yourself that the puppy is as healthy as possible, and then once you make your decision to share your life with a particular puppy, and they are old enough to bring home, make an appointment with your own veterinarian for a complete examination.

However, before you take your new puppy home, there are general signs of good health to be aware of, including the following:

Body Fat – a healthy puppy will look round and well fed, with an obvious layer of fat over their rib cage.

Breathing – a healthy puppy will breathe quietly, without coughing, wheezing or sneezing.

Coat Condition – a healthy puppy will not be itchy and will have a soft coat with no dandruff, dullness, greasiness or bald spots.

Energy Level – a well-rested puppy will be alert and energetic.

Hearing – a healthy puppy should react if you clap your hands or snap your fingers behind their head.

Genitals – a healthy puppy will not have any sort of discharge visible in or around their genital or anal regions.

Mobility – a healthy puppy will walk and run normally without wobbling, limping or seeming to be weak, stiff or sore.

Vision – a healthy puppy will have bright, clear eyes without crust or discharge and they should notice if a ball is rolled past or a toy is tossed within their field of vision.

The Ideal Guardian

Once you have established that you have what it takes to share your life with a dog (by considering the questions in the previous Section), you should consider the following tips to determine whether the Cavapoo would be the right breed for you and your family.

The Cavapoo will be an excellent choice for moderate-energy individuals or families with older children that understand how to respect a dog that is friendly, sweet natured and playful. This dog can also be a good companion for senior adults who have the energy, time and mobility required to provide this companion (that always wants to be with you) with the moderate daily exercise and mental stimulation they need.

Keep in mind that while a well-socialized Cavapoo will usually be accepting of both unknown dogs and humans and generally peaceful with the entire world, when not trained to heed their guardian's lead, they can develop a stubborn streak. While this dog won't often get his or herself into any sort of serious mischief, any dog that is babied too much can develop behavior problems. For instance, it is possible for this sweet dog to become snappish if they think leadership has defaulted to them.

The ideal guardian for the Happy Cavapoo will be a person (or family) who is retired or works at home, and enjoys several moderate energy daily walks and engaging their dog in some time for play at the local park. Also, for those more energetic dogs, a canine sport would be fun for everyone. This guardian will also be aware of this dog's strong desire to always be in close quarters with their humans. Be aware that this dog may develop depression and separation anxiety if they are expected to spend long hours alone every day.

This ideal guardian will also understand the basics of socializing and gentle, fair training, without raised voices, and depending on the energy level of a particular dog, may also enjoy teaching this companion a fun canine sport, or be willing to involve this canine companion in their own moderate daily walking or hiking routine.

As an example, the ideal happy Cavapoo guardian will be someone who works at home or is retired, and takes his or her dog out for a 30-minute walk, so they can empty their bladder and bowels first thing every morning before breakfast, rain or shine.

After returning home, everyone will have their breakfast and then (since you work at home or are retired) your dog can relax on the couch for a couple of hours while you work about the home. Before long it's noon and time to leash up your little shadow companion and head off for another walk. Depending on the weather, you may finish up at a securely fenced local dog park for an off leash fun game of fetch or play with other dogs. If it's a hot day out, always carry water for your dog, and don't let them play too long.

Back home for a midday dental snack for your dog and lunch for you, while you take time (depending on this dog's age) to teach basic commands, play a short game, or maybe teach some tricks before your dog has a snooze and you get back to your time at home.

Now it's about 4:00 pm and again it's time to get you and your dog outside for a 20-30 minute walk, and if it's not too hot or too cold out, perhaps another short play at the park. Keep in mind that if you live where the winters are harsh and you have access to a treadmill, this sturdy little dog can quickly be taught to exercise indoors alongside you on a treadmill.

Also, cold or wet weather will mean that this little dog needs a raincoat or a warm winter coat when walking outside. If snow is involved, since the Cavapoo has very soft hair, the snow may stick to their legs and build up. Do NOT simply pull the snow off, as it will rip their hair out. Take them home and place them in a warm bath to easily melt off any snow accumulation.

Back home and time to prepare dinner for both dog and human, then after dinner (again depending on the age of your dog) perhaps a few more minutes of basic command and/or trick training before you each have some lazy time in front of the fire or TV screen.

Now it's getting to be later evening and before bed you need to put your Cavapoo on leash and take them outside for a quick walk around the block, so they can drain out their bladder before bed.

Everyone now in his or her respective beds as both human and dog have a rejuvenating sleep before the start of the next day when you do this (or something similar) all over again.

Of course, this is just one scenario that would be excellent for the Happy Cavapoo, and with a little imagination on your part, there are many others that would fit the bill quite nicely.

Also, don't forget to check out your local weekend canine sporting facilities, and take the time to get you and your dog involved, because your weekend would be well spent teaching this dog how to run an Agility course, or perhaps participate in Advanced Obedience or even a Freestyle Dance competition.

In a Nutshell

While learning how to choose the right puppy is important, even more important is your ability to ask and honestly answer the questions outlined in this Chapter that will help you to understand if you truly are a good fit for being the ideal guardian for the sweet-natured and friendly Cavapoo, who will be your constant and loyal companion.

Remember that if you don't really have the time, commitment and knowledge necessary to properly socialize and raise this affectionate little dog, you will inevitably end up with an unhappy dog, which will lead to health and behavioral issues, which then will lead to a stressed family, possibly angry neighbors, and extra expenses to hire a professional to help you reverse unwanted behavioral problems.

Chapter 10: Humans Make a LOT of Stupid Mistakes

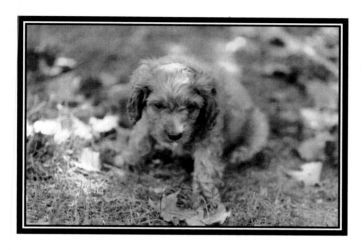

"Heaven goes by favor. If it went by merit,
you would stay out and your dog would go in."
— Mark Twain

Far too often we humans don't even realize we are the cause of creating behavioral problems in our canine companions, and when we're not aware and paying attention, we may be causing a lot of issues that can actually be entirely avoided.

Besides the more obvious problems that can arise with a dog that is bred for tracking, hunting, search and rescue or detection work and can become a unhappy member of your family when not raised properly and engaged in a working capacity, there are many other situations or unwanted outcomes that may arise that can be avoided.

For instance, not taking the time to properly socialize your Cavapoo, forgetting about desensitizing them to loud noises, falling prey to those pleading eyes that this little character knows how to work to their own advantage (especially when food is around), feeding too much, not exercising enough, accidentally rewarding them at the wrong time, or not taking the time to teach basic rules and boundaries, can all lead to plenty of trouble in later life and create unhappiness and unwanted behavior and health issues that could have been avoided.

As well, not being aware of the adolescent craziness time in a young dog's life and how to get through it, and many other less obvious mistakes, such as choosing the wrong collar or leash, sleeping in your bed, or free feeding can all result in the creation of problems.

While we humans may be well meaning, besides the obvious disasters that we can create when we don't properly train or socialize our canine friends, we can inadvertently make a lot of stupid mistakes when raising our canine companions that will cause our fur friends to needlessly suffer.

Let's begin with the more obvious *"Preventing Socialization Behavioral Issues"* that can lead to problems later in life, and proceed further into areas of *"Accidental Rewards"* that may not be so obvious, then touch upon *"Basic Rules and Boundaries"* and *"Adolescent Craziness",* and finish this chapter with *"Less Obvious Stupid Human Mistakes".*

Preventing Socialization Behavioral Issues

In order to prevent behavioral issues you first need to be aware of how easy it is to inadvertently create them yourself.

Much of how your Cavapoo learns to behave will depend entirely upon you, how extensively they were socialized as a puppy and how much they are continually being socialized throughout their life.

Without proper socialization, even the most naturally friendly dog, like the Cavapoo, can become neurotic, unsociable and learn to act out aggressively toward unknown dogs, smaller animals or people. This is a situation that can get a small dog deemed nasty or even dangerous should they act out aggressively for any reason.

Many people don't realize how important it is to properly and continually socialize their dogs, even small ones like the Cavapoo, in several different areas, because without proper socialization, many behavioral problems could become a daily occurrence.

Never make the mistake of thinking that you only need to socialize your Cavapoo puppy during the first few months of their life and that they will then be fine for the rest of their life, because all dogs require constant socializing.

As well, once they reach adolescence, their personality can really begin to assert itself, and this is when, without constant and vigilant daily socializing and training, any aggressive or anti-social tendencies may begin to erupt.

Generally speaking, the majority of an adult dog's habits and behavioral traits will be formed between the ages of birth and one year of age. While it is even more important to introduce puppies to a wide variety of sights, sounds, smells and situations during the most formative period in their young life, which is usually their first 16 weeks, all dogs, no matter their age, need to be exposed to different people, dogs, animals, places and unusual sights and sounds throughout their entire adult life.

Socializing With Unknown Dogs

Any dog, despite their natural personality, that is not regularly socialized may become shy, nervous or suspicious around unfamiliar or unusual dogs, animals, people or circumstances, which could lead to nervous or fearful behavior, which can then lead to aggression.

Daily on-leash dog walks are great opportunities for your Cavapoo to see and possibly meet other dogs and different people, as well as practice proper behavior when out and about.

Remember to take it slowly and never put your dog in a situation where he or she feels uncomfortable or feels forced into being around other canines. Your dog should always be given the option to walk away, with lots of space.

When socializing a young puppy, remember to introduce him or her first to the *more calm and friendlier* of dogs, because introducing your pup to a dog that may be overly boisterous or not so friendly with other dogs may result in a negative experience. Negative experiences at a young age may later result in a fear of other dogs. I would suggest finding a local puppy class with around 8-10 other puppies, so that you can carefully supervise socializing and guided play.

Socializing With Unknown People

Proper socialization also means taking your puppy (or dog) everywhere with you and introducing them to many different people of all ages, sizes and ethnicities, so they will learn what is normal and acceptable in their daily life.

Remember – do NOT get into the habit of always carrying this small dog when he or she is a puppy. They need to walk on their own feet so that they don't develop unwanted behavior problems, such as *"armpit alligator"* tendencies (snapping when someone stops to say hello) that can result from being in an elevated position where they feel they must protect their human.

Also important, will be getting your puppy or dog used to the noise and unpredictable actions of young children. You will want to closely supervise play, so that children are not accidentally being too rough or screaming in high-pitched voices, because this can be very frightening for a sensitive young puppy or dog that is unfamiliar with children.

Be especially careful when introducing your puppy to young children who may accidentally hurt your puppy, because you don't want your dog to become fearful of children as this could lead to aggression issues later on in life.

Environmental Socialization

It can be a BIG mistake not to take the time to introduce your Cavapoo puppy to a wide variety of different environments, because when they are not comfortable with different sights, smells and sounds, this could cause them (and you) stress and trauma later in their adult life.

Be creative and take your puppy everywhere you can imagine when they are young, so that no matter where they travel, whether strolling along a noisy city sidewalk or beside a peaceful shoreline, they will be equally comfortable. Also, don't forget to train this dog to like travelling inside their very useful Sherpa bag.

Do not make the mistake of only taking your puppy into areas where you live and will frequently travel, because they need to also be comfortable visiting areas you might not often visit, such as noisy construction sites, airports or a shopping area across town.

Your puppy needs to see all sorts of sights, sounds and situations so that they will not become fearful, should they need to travel with you outside of their immediate neighbourhood.

Your Cavapoo will take their cues from you, which means that when you are calm and in control of every situation, they will learn to be the same because they will trust and calmly follow your lead.

For instance, take them to a noisy construction site, to the airport where they can watch people and hear planes landing and taking off, to a local park where they can see a baseball game, for a stroll beside a schoolyard at recess time when noisy children are out playing, or to the local zoo or farm and let them get a close up look at horses, pigs and ducks. Use your imagination.

Again, never think that socialization is something that only takes place when your Cavapoo is a young puppy, as proper socialization is on-going for your dog's entire life.

Fear of Loud Noises

Many dogs can show extreme fear of loud noises, such as fireworks, sirens, thunderstorms or home security alarms, especially dogs that are more sensitive, such as the Cavapoo. We humans need to learn how to either prevent this trauma in the first place or learn how to appropriately respond to a dog that is afraid of loud noises.

When you take the time to desensitize your dog to these types of noises when they are very young, it will be much easier on them during stormy weather, holidays such as Halloween or New Year's, when fireworks are often a part of the festivities, when an ambulance or fire truck roars past with sirens wailing, or when your fire or security alarm is activated.

Desensitization Devices: there are several ways you can help to desensitize your Cavapoo, so that they are not fearful of high-pitched alarms, and loud, popping noises, including the following:

CDs: you can purchase CD's that are a collection of unusual sounds, such as vacuums or hoovers, airplanes, sirens, smoke alarms, fireworks, people clapping hands, screaming children, and more (or you can easily make your own), that you can play while working in your kitchen or relaxing in your living room or lounge.

When you play these sounds and pretend that everything is normal, the next time your puppy or dog hears these types of sounds elsewhere, they will not become upset or agitated because they have learned to ignore them.

Bubble Wrap: is also another simple way to desensitize a Cavapoo that is fearful of unexpected sounds. Show them the bubble wrap, pop a few of the cells and if they do not run away, give them a treat. You can start with the bubble wrap that has small, quieter cells, and then graduate them to the larger celled (louder) bubble wrap. You can also take things even farther by blowing up some small paper bags or balloons and loudly popping them in front of your dog, or taking them to the rifle range.

Thunder Shirts: some dogs will respond well to wearing a *"Thunder Shirt"*, which is specifically designed to alleviate anxiety or trauma associated with loud rumbling, popping or banging noises. The idea behind the design of the Thunder Shirt is that the gentle pressure it creates is similar to a hug that, for some dogs, has a calming effect.

Relaxation Collars: there are basically two types of collars designed to help relax or calm an upset puppy or dog. One uses scent or calming pheromones, while the other uses species-specific music at appropriate decibel levels to calm a fearful or stressed dog.

TV or Radio: sometimes all that is required to calm a dog that is stressed by loud noises is to play your inside TV or Radio station with the sounds of relaxing music, louder than you might normally, to help disguise the exterior noise of fireworks or thunder.

Always be aware that some dogs literally lose their minds and do things that make no logical sense when they hear the loud popping or screeching noises of fireworks and various alarms and start trembling, running or trying to hide and you cannot communicate with them at all.

Make certain that your dog cannot harm itself trying to escape from these types of noises, and if possible, calmly hold them until they begin to relax.

For instance, my dog, Boris, used to try and escape through the drain in the bathtub (go figure), because loud popping noises literally caused him to lose his mind.

Make sure that YOU are acting appropriately yourself, by not panicking or having weak, *"feeling sorry"* or *"angry and frustrated"* energy around an upset dog, because this will only make matters worse. When the person who is supposed to be your dog's support system is also feeling weak or acting unstable, your dog will have nowhere to turn. Instead, support them by pretending that nothing is wrong and if you must talk to them, do so in a calm, yet assertive voice.

Never underestimate the importance of taking the time to continually (not just when they are puppies) socialize and desensitize your Cavapoo puppy to all manner of sounds, because to do so will make everyone happier in the future and will be teaching them to be a calm and well-balanced member of your family in every situation.

Accidental Rewards

Many times, we humans are guilty of accidentally rewarding our puppies and dogs for engaging in types of behavior we are not happy with, and the following are some of the more obvious things we may be doing that are inadvertently rewarding, and thus encouraging, an unwanted behavior.

Aggression Rewards

Many people unknowingly get into the habit of accidentally rewarding their puppies or dogs for displaying nervousness, fear, barking, growling or lunging at another dog or person by picking them up, talking soothingly, or offering them a treat. I see this happen all too often.

While most of these habits are not generally something a friendly Cavapoo is known for engaging in, should you accidentally reward your dog when they are displaying any sort of unbalanced energy, this actually turns out to be a reward for them, and you will be teaching them to continue with this type of unwanted behavior.

As well, picking up a small dog or puppy when they are growling, barking or acting out inappropriately, again rewards them and places them in a top dog position where they literally have just gained the higher ground.

A dog in the *"top dog"* position feels more confident and, depending on your energy, will usually then become more dominant than the person or dog they may have just growled at when they were at *"ground level"*.

Rather than accidentally rewarding your Cavapoo for displaying unwanted behavior, the correct action to take in such a situation is to gently correct your puppy or dog with firm yet calm energy (that is just a little stronger than the energy your dog is displaying) by distracting them with a firm *"No!"* and a quick sideways snap of the leash to get their attention back on you, so that they learn to let you deal with whatever situation has caused them to react badly.

If you allow a fearful, nervous or shy dog to deal with situations that unnerve them and cause them to act out aggressively when they encounter unfamiliar circumstances, you will have created a problem that could escalate into something very serious.

The same is true of situations where a young puppy may feel the need to protect itself from a larger or older dog that may come charging in for a sniff or is acting confrontational. It's the human guardian's responsibility to protect their puppy or dog, so that they do not feel that they must react with fear or aggression in order to protect his or herself or the human at the other end of the leash.

No matter the age or size of your Cavapoo puppy or dog, allowing them to display aggression or any sort of unwanted behavior toward another dog, animal or person is never a laughing matter and this type of behavior must be immediately curtailed.

Excitement Rewards

It's important to recognize that attention paid to an overly excited or out-of-control puppy or dog, even negative attention, is likely going to be rewarding for your fur friend. If your dog is not receiving enough of your attention, they will quickly learn to do whatever it takes to get the attention they desire.

Bottom line, when you engage with an out-of-control puppy or dog, you end up actually rewarding them for acting out in an unstable manner, and encouraging them to continue with more overly exuberant behavior you might not be very pleased about.

Be careful that you're not teaching your dog to act out with crazy energy every time they see you.

For instance, chasing after a puppy when they have taken something they are not supposed to have, picking them up when they are barking or showing aggression, pushing them off when they jump on you or other people, or yelling when they refuse to come when called, are all forms of attention that can actually be rewarding and cause more of the same behavior.

Instead, remain calm and assertive and be consistent with your training, so that your dog learns how to control their energy and play quietly and appropriately without jumping on everyone or engaging in barking or mouthy behavior.

Interaction Rewards

If your Cavapoo displays excited energy simply from being petted by you, or anyone else, you will need to teach yourself, your family and your friends to ignore your fur friend until he or she calms down. Otherwise, you will be inadvertently teaching your canine companion that the touch of humans means excitement, and this behavioral problem will continue to escalate.

For instance, when you continue to engage with your overly excited puppy or dog, you are actually rewarding them for out-of-control behavior and literally teaching them that when they see humans, you want them to display excited energy.

Too many people encourage their dog to be nuts, for instance, when they return home and greet their dog in a highly excited state. While it's nice to know that your dog is happy to see you, when you forget about being your dog's calm pack leader just a few times, this may be enough to send your dog the message that they can no longer rely upon you to be their leader, and that seeing humans means they must now display out-of-control excitement.

Instead, when you come home, greet your dog calmly and quietly, and if they are at all excited, do NOT touch or talk to them until they calm down. Otherwise, your dog will learn that humans are a source of excitement, and long, consistently vigilant work on your part (with help from your friends and family) will be the only way to reverse this unwanted behavior.

Another thing to keep in mind is that children are often a source of high energy and excitement that can cause a puppy or dog to quickly become extremely wound up.

If you don't want to create an on-going behavioral problem, that could accidentally get someone injured, you will need to be very vigilant about NOT permitting young children to engage with an excited puppy or dog.

Important Basic Rules and Boundaries

You can prevent many future behavioral problems when you take the time to ensure that your Cavapoo learns basic rules and boundaries. All that's necessary for effectively teaching your puppy (or dog) these basics is a calm, consistent and firm approach, combined with your endless patience.

Basic rules and boundaries would include things such as:

- no dogs allowed in the kitchen when preparing food
- no begging at the human's dinner table
- humans through the door first
- no sleeping in the human bed
- no raiding the garbage can
- no jumping up on tables or counters
- no helping yourself to *"tootsie rolls"* from the cat's litter box
- no chasing the neighbor's cat

Many puppies are ready to begin basic training at about 10 to 12 weeks of age, and some will be ready at 8 weeks. However, be careful not to overdo it when they are less than four months of age, as their attention span may be short.

With younger puppies, make your training sessions no more than 5 or 10 minutes, positive and pleasant with plenty of praise and/or treats, so that your puppy will be looking forward to their next session.

Also, begin to introduce hand signals that go along with the verbal commands so that once they learn both, you can remove the verbal commands in favor of just hand signals.

Consistently teach your puppy or dog the *All Important Three*, which is the "Come", "Sit" and "Stay" commands (more about this in Chapter 12: Training Basics For a Happy Cavapoo), and use them every day in every opportunity to help your young dog progress through their unpredictable adolescent period.

Adolescent Craziness

Too often, we humans become impatient and frustrated and give up on our dogs when they transition from being the cute, cuddly and mostly obedient little puppy they once were and become all kinds of craziness.

Instead of riding the adolescent storm, it is often during this confusing and trying adolescent stage of a dog's life that they end up behind bars when the humans who promised to love and protect them, abandon their once happy fur friend at the local SPCA or rescue facility.

With consistency, understanding, the right information, and endless patience and perseverance, you and your fur friend can emerge out the other side of this adolescent period with a much stronger bond.

Firstly, you need to know that not all dogs go through an intensely crazy adolescent period. Secondly, when you remain consistent with your socializing and training during this time, you can live through puppy adolescence and come out the other side a much more knowledgeable and patient guardian.

Remember, you've already lived through potty training, teething, socializing and basic rules and boundaries with your young Cavapoo, and you need to feel proud of all your accomplishments and the leaps and bounds you and your puppy have accomplished together over the last several months.

If your adolescent dog is beginning to act out and push your buttons, rather than giving up on them, it's time to remain calm, consistent and persistent, and re-visit basic rules and boundaries, while keeping in mind that you will eventually be able to enjoy the happy rewards that all those months of diligent puppy training have brought to your relationship.

During adolescence, you may experience several changes in your dog's personality that you're not exactly pleased about. For instance, your young Cavapoo may:

- no longer be as friendly with strangers

- start to show their stubborn side
- ignore you when called
- appear to have suddenly gone deaf
- ignore the basic commands they've already learned
- start to relieve themselves inside again
- bark or cry when left alone
- begin to mark territory
- refuse to go walking in the rain

Welcome to the world of canine adolescence, where it appears that all your previous work was for naught and your puppy has turned into some sort of monster.

Don't panic, because every dog is different and your dog's adolescent period may go by without notice. However, being prepared for the worst will help you ride any impending storm and get you both safely out the other side where you can enjoy an even closer relationship than you previously had.

The adolescent phase may be very subtle for your puppy or on the other hand, it may be so dramatic that frustration with your fur friend is becoming a daily occurrence.

If frustration is getting the upper hand, rather than letting it get worse, consider the benefits of hiring a professional, who can provide insight and valuable assistance to help you through this stage of your puppy's development.

<u>Less Obvious Stupid Human Mistakes</u>

There are many less obvious mistakes we humans can inadvertently make with our dogs that can also lead to behavioral problems later in life, some of which include:

Sleeping in Your Bed: many people make the mistake of allowing a crying puppy to sleep with them in their bed. While this may help to calm and comfort a new puppy, it will set a dangerous precedent that can result in behavioral problems later in their life, plus a sleeping human body could easily crush a tiny puppy.

As much as it may pull on your heart strings to hear your new puppy crying the first couple of nights in their kennel, a little tough love at the beginning will keep them safe while helping them to learn to both love and respect you as their leader.

Picking Them Up at the Wrong Time: never pick your puppy up if they display nervousness, fear or aggression (such as growling) toward an object, person or other pet, because this will be rewarding them for unbalanced behavior.

Instead, your puppy needs to be gently corrected by you, with firm and calm energy, so that they learn not to react with fear or aggression.

Armpit Alligators: when your Cavapoo is a small size, be aware that many guardians get into the bad habit of carrying a small dog or puppy far too much.

Remember that they need to be on the ground and walking on their own, so that they do not become overly confident because a dog that is carried by their guardian is literally being placed in the *"top dog"* position.

Be aware that humans who constantly carry small dogs or puppies, rather than allowing them to walk on their own, can often inadvertently create what I refer to as an *"armpit alligator"* situation. This is where you see someone carrying a cute little dog and you stop to say hello, only to be greeted by snapping jaws and sharp teeth.

Even dogs that are friendly and not naturally wary or suspicious of strangers, such as the Cavapoo, can learn to become intolerant if they don't receive adequate socialization, which means that it is always possible to allow them to become protective or possessive of *"their"* humans.

Playing Too Hard or Too Long: many humans play too hard or allow their children to play too long or too roughly with their puppy. You need to remember that your young puppy tires very easily and especially during the critical growing phases of their young life, they need their rest.

Hand Play: always discourage your puppy from chewing or biting your hands, or any part of your body for that matter.

Do NOT get into the habit of playing the *"hand"* game, where you rough up your puppy and slide them across the floor with your hands, because this will teach them that your hands are playthings and you will have to work hard to break this bad habit.

When my puppy came home with me at 10-weeks of age, the breeder had already been playing the hand game and it took me a very long time to teach my Boris that biting human hands was not acceptable behavior. Interestingly, when he sees people that he has not seen for years, that he used to know when he was a young puppy, this old habit often re-surfaces for a short while.

When your puppy is teething, they will naturally want to chew on everything within reach, and this will include you. As cute as you might think it is, this is not an acceptable behavior and you need to gently, but firmly, discourage the habit.

A light flick with a finger on the end of your puppy nose, combined with a firm "NO" and removing the enticing fingers by making a fist when they are trying to bite human fingers, will discourage them from this activity.

Not Getting Used to Grooming: not taking the time to get your Cavapoo used to a regular grooming routine, including bathing, brushing, toenail clipping and teeth brushing, can lead to a lifetime of trauma for both human and dog every time these procedures must be performed.

Set aside a few minutes each day for your grooming routine.

NOTE: get your puppy used to being up high on a table or countertop when you are grooming them. This way, when it comes time for a full grooming session or a visit to the vet's office, where they will be placed on an examination table, they will not be stressed because this will already be a familiar situation.

Free Feeding: means to keep food in your puppy's bowl 24/7, so that they can eat any time of the day or night, whenever they feel like it.

While free feeding a young puppy can be a good idea (especially with very small dogs), until they are about four or five months old, many guardians often get into the bad habit of allowing their adult dogs to continue to eat food any time they want, by leaving food out 24/7.

The Cavapoo is not especially food motivated and will usually walk away when they are full, and may not eat food that is left out. However, every dog is different, so don't get into the habit of leaving food out 24/7 because (a) they no longer associate you being in control of the food, and (b) if your particular dog gets used to eating too much, they will quickly gain weight and become obese.

Getting into this type of habit can be a serious mistake, as your dog is not a cat, and needs to know that you are absolutely in control of their food.

Treating Them Like Children: do not get into the bad habit of treating your dog like a small, furry human; even though they may try their best to please you and their doggy smarts could help them to succeed in most instances, not honoring them for the amazing dog they are will only cause them confusion that could lead to behavioral problems.

IMPORTANT: remember that the one thing your dog is the absolute BEST at, is **Being a Dog**.

A well-balanced dog thrives on rules and boundaries, and when they understand that there is no question that you are their leader and they are your follower, they will live a contented, happy and stress-free life.

Distraction and Replacement: when your puppy tries to chew on your hand, foot, clothing, or anything else that is not fair game, you need to firmly and calmly tell them "No", and then distract them by replacing what they are not supposed to be chewing with something they <u>are</u> permitted to chew, such as an appropriate toy.

Make sure that you happily praise them every time they choose the toy to chew on. If your puppy persists in chewing on you, remove yourself from the equation by getting up and walking away. If they are really persistent, put them inside their kennel with a favorite chew toy until they calm down.

Always praise your puppy when they stop inappropriate behavior or replace inappropriate behavior with something that is acceptable to you, so that they begin to understand what they can and cannot do.

Flat Collar Nightmares

Many humans simply don't realize how important it is to choose the "right" kind of collar for their canine companion. Add this to the fact that there is an ever-increasing array of tempting colors and styles to choose from and it's very easy to get distracted and forget about choosing what you really need for your dog.

What you really need in a collar is one that will also keep your Cavapoo safe and secure. While the flat collar may be fine for a calm dog that never pulls, leaps about or suddenly tries to do an about face and take off running in a different direction to chase that teasing squirrel or taunting cat, this is not a very safe reality.

Of course, while you will choose what you will for your dog, after 40 some years of working with dogs and experiencing possibly every type of terrifying, unexpected disaster while out walking a dog, the ONLY collar I feel absolutely confident using (because I know that the dog I'm in control of cannot wiggle out of it), is the "Martingale" collar.

Flat collars, unless you have them cinched up so tight that you're almost cutting off your dog's air supply, can be fairly easy for most dogs to get out of.

All dogs are amazing athletes, and even though you may have a firm grip on that leash, they can back away from you, wiggle, twist and contort themselves in a quick instant, flip their head and the collar is off – bye, bye doggy!

The Martingale Collar

There are several reasons why the Martingale dog collar is far superior to a flat collar:

- comfortable for your dog to wear
- safe because your dog cannot wiggle out of it
- best training collar

The Martingale collar looks much the same as a flat collar, with one very important difference – there is a triangular piece of chain in the middle of it. This chain is attached to the collar with two rings, with a third ring in the middle of the chain, which is where you attach your leash.

When there is no tension on the collar (from them pulling on the leash), the collar hangs loose and comfortable. However, when there IS tension on the collar, that little piece of chain tightens so that your dog cannot get out of their collar.

My dog (despite his short nose) has been wearing the same Martingale "training" collar for over 14 years and will continue to do so, because this collar conveys important messages between my dog and myself.

That little piece of triangular chain makes a slight noise when you sharply tug it, and this sends a message to your dog that you want their attention on you. It's simply the best collar for teaching your dog to walk calmly by your side and to remind them that YOU are in charge.

When buying a Martingale collar for your Cavapoo, take him or her with you because it needs to be the correct size to fit over the widest part of their head. Then, once you've got the right size for your dog, you need to pay strict attention to the <u>correct way to</u> <u>adjust</u> the collar for maximum effect and safety.

Adjusting the Martingale Collar: once you've placed the collar over your dog's head, you need to adjust the length so that when you attach the leash to the outside ring and pull it tight, when the two inside rings come together, there is still a gap between these two rings of approximately two human finger widths. You never want the two inside rings to touch.

You can now enjoy comfortable and safe walks with your Happy Cavapoo companion.

Flexi-Leash Fiasco

Personally, flexi, retractable or extendable dog leashes are high on my list of pet peeves, for several important reasons, because they:

- are dangerous for human and dog alike
- allow the dog to be in the wrong walking position
- allow the humans to forget their responsibilities
- are difficult to securely grip
- are an excuse for not properly training your dog
- can accidentally break

While many people believe that a retractable leash is a good way to allow their dogs more freedom to roam while still keeping them securely attached, the above reasons highlight why these leashes can be a very bad idea. See below for more details.

Injury to human and dog: these leashes are usually spring-loaded, many feet long (usually 26 feet or 7.9 meters), and thin cords wound up inside a cumbersome plastic compartment with a handle and a button to control how much of the leash is extended.

As you can imagine, it's far more difficult to control a dog that is roaming about 20 or more feet away from you, than it would be if they were attached to a standard 4 to 6 foot leash.

If your dog gets used to having a 20-foot (6 meter) or more leeway, they will be busy sniffing interesting scents, and can quickly run out into traffic, be surprised by another dog rushing in, or get tangled up with a person and a dog, which can cause both injury to the dogs and people, or may cause a fight between the two dogs.

These leashes are also serious tripping hazards that can cause many injuries.

For instance, the daughter of one of my dog whispering clients broke her toe as a result of tripping over a flexi-leash, I have suffered painful "rope" burns several times, and once was hit in the head (ouch!) with the hard and heavy plastic handle as it snapped back when the person holding it lost their grip and dropped it.

In addition, every flexi or retractable leash is equipped with a brake to stop the unwinding of the cord at various lengths. If your dog is running and all of a sudden comes to the end of their freedom, unless you drop the handle, they will be forced to come to a very abrupt stop that can injure a dog's neck or spine.

Incorrect Walking Position: the ONLY place your dog should ever be when you're out walking is beside you, and when you allow them to freely roam 20 or more feet from wherever you are, besides being lax about teaching your dog the correct walking position, you are *"telling"* them that you are no longer in charge. A dog that believes they are in charge can get you BOTH into a lot of trouble.

Forgetting Your Human Responsibilities: when you're out walking with your puppy or dog, as their leader, you are responsible for everything they do, including picking up after them. A retractable leash allows your dog to literally be out of your sight. While you're busy chatting with a neighbor or checking your phone messages, who knows what sort of *"message"* your dog may be depositing in the neighbor's yard.

You can be fined for not picking up after your dog, not to mention gaining yourself a bad reputation from your neighbors or other more responsible dog walkers.

Difficult to Securely Grip: the flexi leash has a large, cumbersome handle that is quite slippery and difficult to securely hold onto. If your companion suddenly lunges or changes direction, the chances of you losing your grip are quite high, and when that happens, the consequences can be dangerously grave.

Once dropped, your dog is now dragging a bouncing, loudly clattering handle, which can be very noisy on a sidewalk or hard surface.

This very thing has happened to me in a busy, high traffic area, when walking someone else's dog, and I can tell you from first-hand experience that this is a highly stressful and frightening situation I would not want to wish on anyone.

Unless your dog has been trained to remain calmly sitting while rifles are fired near their head, this flexi leash that seems to be chasing them can be a very scary experience that will cause most dogs to run.

When your dog is scared, they will run even faster, while you run after them adding to the chaos with your panic-stricken screams to stop before they get killed trying to cross a busy intersection. Not a good scene.

Poor Training: while many might believe they are giving their dog more freedom by using a retractable leash, they are actually missing out on properly training their dog to heel beside them and to respond appropriately to the all-important "come" or "recall" command.

The very nature of a flexi leash is such that the dog is often out in front of the person who is supposed to be in charge, and always *"pulling"*, which to an approaching dog can look like an aggressive stance, resulting in the other dog thinking he or she must retaliate with a defensive stance. All of this, as you can imagine, has the potential to result in a scuffle between dogs and humans.

Accidental Breakage: there is a great deal of wear on a small diameter cord that is constantly unwinding and rewinding and you may not notice a worn area until it actually breaks. Then, you've got a potential runaway dog disaster to hopefully recover from, before the dog gets severely injured or killed by a vehicle, or finds his or herself in some other type of serious trouble.

Improve your training, have better control, make your life easier, avoid injuries, and ensure the safety and security of yourself and your furry best friend by choosing a Martingale collar and a standard 4-foot leash.

Sled Dog Fiasco

One last thought about what I call the *"Sled Dog Fiasco"*. Many people think that buying a harness is a better choice than the proper collar for their canine companion. However, the only time a harness is actually the right choice is if you have a strong sled dog that you need to put in harness, so that they can pull you.

What happens when you put a dog such as a Cavapoo in a harness is that (1) they are automatically in the wrong walking position, being head and shoulders in front of you; (2) you no longer have control of their head and cannot correct unwanted behavior; and (3) they now are in control of you and are much more powerful and potentially difficult to control, because the entire weight and strength of their body is attached to that harness.

Take Away Tip: *"Harnesses are for sled dogs"*.

In a Nutshell

It cannot be emphasized strongly enough how important it is to properly socialize your Cavapoo puppy, and understand that we humans often unknowingly reward our dogs at the wrong time, which can actually cause behavioral issues later in life.

Re-visit this Chapter information and think about what other mistakes you may be inadvertently making, so that you can do your best to avoid simple mistakes we humans often are guilty of making with our dogs, that can lead to an unhappy dog that suffers from behavioral problems later in life.

Also, when training your puppy or dog, keep in mind that the type of leash and collar you choose can make a big difference.

Chapter 11: Happy Cavapoo Body Language

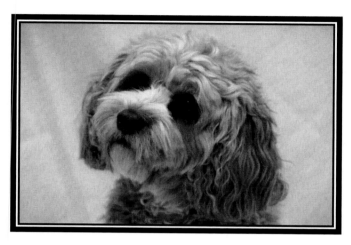

*"Money can buy a fine dog, but
only love can make him wag his tail."*
— Kinky Friedman

We all know good communication is not just about the words we use. Our tone of voice, energy and our body language help to package up and deliver our meaning every day. While most people can effectively communicate their thoughts and feelings through words, we need to generally be reliant upon reading our dog's body language in order to know if they are happy or sad.

Because our dogs don't speak our language, the only way to truly comprehend and communicate with them is for us to understand and appreciate what they are telling us through their body and vocal language.

Often, gestures or actions that we assume mean one thing are actually the dog telling us the exact opposite, and determining what that wagging tail or barking really means can sometimes be the difference between a belly rub and a bite.

How happy would you be if you could not communicate with your family at home? Would you develop behaviour issues over time? Of course you would, and the same is also true for your beloved dog.

They need you to understand what they are "telling you" and how they feel, in order to be a happy family member. For instance, learning to properly "read" your dog's intentions can easily prevent an unwanted encounter during a visit to the local park.

Therefore, taking the time to educate yourself about basic canine body language and paying attention to your dog's body language (including their face, posture, barking and tail position) is an important prerequisite for raising a content and well-behaved dog.

This Chapter will teach you exactly that – to understand the basics of what your furry friend (and those dogs around you) are trying to "tell" you and how they feel, so that you can share a happy lifelong partnership together.

So, don't wait and read on.

What's With All the Wagging and Barking?

While a well-socialized Cavapoo may often happily wag their tail, it can be a mistake to automatically assume that if your dog, or someone else's dog, is wagging their tail, they are happy and friendly.

What Does the Wag Mean?

When determining a dog's true intent or demeanor, it's important to take into consideration the complete dog posture, rather than just the tail, because it's entirely possible that a dog can be wagging his or her tail just before it decides to take an aggressive lunge toward you or your dog.

More important in determining the emotional state of most dogs is the height or positioning of their tail. For instance, a tail that is held parallel to your dog's back usually suggests that they are feeling relaxed, whereas if the tail is held stiffly vertical, this usually means that they may be feeling aggressive or dominant.

Also keep in mind that certain dog tails are carried differently for different reasons. Depending on which dog tail, you will have more or less visible cues. The opposite is also true of other dogs reading your dog's body language, because a dog with a docked or curled tail can sometimes send confusing messages to others.

A tail held much lower can mean that your dog is feeling stressed, afraid, submissive or unwell and if the tail is tucked underneath the dog's body, this is most often a sign that the dog is feeling highly stressed, nervous, fearful or threatened by another dog or person.

Paying attention to your dog's tail (and any dog tails around you) can help you to know when you need to step in and make some space between your dog and another, more dominant dog.

Of course, different breeds naturally carry their tails at different heights, some dogs have tightly curled tails and some dogs don't have any visible tails. So, you will need to take this into consideration so that you get used to their particular body language signals.

As well, the speed at which the tail is moving will give you an idea of the mental state of your dog, because the speed of the wag usually indicates how excited a dog may be.

For instance, a slow, slightly swinging wag can often mean that a dog is tentative about greeting another dog, and this is more of a questioning type of wag, whereas a fast-moving tail held high can mean that your dog is about to challenge or threaten another less dominant dog.

Also, a stalking stance, where your dog has raised hackles (hair along the back), lowers their head and slowly creeps forward with an intense stare often happens just before a serious attack. There is also a similar-looking *"play"* stance, and without practice, you may have difficulty identifying the difference between the two.

As an example, I've been sworn at after politely letting a guardian of a larger dog, who was unaware (and didn't want to know) that their dog was stalking my smaller dog and about to do him harm, so be careful how you approach these situations.

What Does the Bark Mean?

Of course, our dogs bark for a wide variety of reasons, and every dog is different, depending upon their natural breed tendencies and how they were raised. The Cavapoo is not a big barker, but when they DO bark, it can be a very loud and shrill sound. This section discusses some of the more common reasons why a dog might be barking.

Communication: since the very first dog, they have communicated over long distances by howling to one another and when in closer proximity, barking to warn off other dogs approaching what they consider to be their territory, or in excitement or happiness when greeting another member of the dog pack.

Now, our domesticated dogs have learned that barking for a wide variety of reasons, such as when alerting us to someone approaching the home, in anticipation of their favorite food, when they are afraid, frustrated or bored, or to let us know they want to play, is an effective way to get the attention of us humans because barking is a loud and difficult noise to ignore.

Danger: many dogs will bark to alert us to visitors or intruders, and we need to learn how to understand the difference between what our dogs perceive as danger and what is truly dangerous, or indeed how to teach our best friends the difference?

We want our dogs to tell us when there is real, imminent danger and in this case, should the danger involve an unwanted intruder, we want them to bark loudly to possibly scare this threat away.

When our dogs are barking for a reason we are not yet aware of, we need to calmly assess the situation rather than immediately becoming annoyed.

We also need to remember that a Cavapoo's sense of smell, hearing and sometimes eyesight is far more acute than our own, which means that we need to give them an opportunity to tell us if they just heard, saw or sensed something that they are worried or uncertain about.

Rather than ignoring our dogs (or yelling at them) when they are attempting to *"tell"* us that something is bothering them, even if we ourselves understand that the noise the dog just heard is only the neighbor's kids coming home from school or a postal delivery, we need to respond appropriately.

We need to <u>calmly</u> acknowledge our dog's concern by saying, *"OK, good dog,"* and then ask them to come to you. This way you have quietly and calmly let your dog know that the situation is nothing to be concerned about and you have asked them to move away from the target they are concerned about, which places you in control, and which will usually stop the barking.

Attention: many dogs will learn to bark to get their owner's attention, just because they are bored or want to be taken outside for an interesting walk or a trip to the local park to chase a ball.

Our canine companions are very good at manipulating us in this way, and if we fall for it, we are setting up an annoying precedent that could plague us for the remainder of our relationship.

For instance, I shared my life with a Blue Heeler who would go berserk with loud barking every time we drove near a park or when we arrived at a park. Even so, I would never reward him for barking, because as annoying and hard on the eardrums as it was, I had to sit calmly inside the vehicle until he stopped barking. If I had let him immediately bound out of the vehicle, I would have inadvertently taught my dog that barking got him exactly what he wanted.

When a dog is barking to gain their guardian's attention, for whatever reason, before we immediately capitulate, first we need to calmly ask our dog to do something for us. After our dog has performed a calm and quiet task for us, such as sit or lie down, then we can decide to give our dog our undivided attention on our terms.

Often you will see a dog and their guardian at the local dog park playing fetch and when the human is not throwing that ball quickly enough to satisfy the dog's desire to run and fetch, the dog will be madly barking at the guardian. This is the equivalent of being sworn at in doggy language.

Don't make the mistake of allowing your puppy or dog to manipulate you in this situation, because if you do, you will soon create a bad habit that will very quickly become not just annoying to you, but also annoying to everyone else at the park.

Before throwing a ball or Frisbee for a dog that loves to retrieve, it's important to always ask the dog to sit and make eye contact with you.

Often the types of canines that are overly exuberant with chasing a ball or Frisbee have learned this barking behavior from their humans, who allowed themselves to be literally at the beck and call of their dog, and created this irritating habit by throwing the ball every time the dog barked.

In this situation, if you allow your dog to dictate to you when you will throw the ball, they will quickly learn that barking gets them their desired result, and you have just created an annoying, rude dog who is yelling at you in doggy language to do their bidding.

In this type of ball-retrieving scenario, the dog has become ball *"obsessed"* and is no longer really paying attention to the guardian's commands, as they are solely focusing on where the ball is.

While there are many situations in which your Cavapoo may bark to convey that they've heard a noise, in all other situations where the barking is done to demand attention, a toy or an object or food, this is when you need to ask them to do something for you, and then only if you want to give them what they are asking for, do you follow through.

As an example, I once had a client whose dog would start to loudly bark and howl every time she left the house to go grocery shopping or pick up the kids from school. This was big time annoying to everyone, not to mention the neighbors, and all of this could have been avoided if the family had taken the time to properly train this dog to be alone for short periods of time when the dog was a young pup.

Bottom line, remember to stay calm when your cute puppy is demanding attention, because even negative attention can be rewarding for your dog, and can lead down a future, unwanted path where he or she will learn further habits that will not be particularly endearing for the human side of the relationship when the cute puppy has become an adult.

Boredom or Separation Anxiety: many dogs, especially those who have not been properly trained or that have not been allowed to understand that they have rules and boundaries and are treated like children, will sharply bark when left at home and are bored or are feeling the anxiety of being alone.

Many times, we humans believe that our dog is barking when being left alone, because he is experiencing *"separation anxiety"*, when in fact what the dog is really experiencing is the frustration of observing a member of the pack which they believe to be their follower (i.e. You) leaving them.

This can happen when you are not a strong enough leader for your playful, little Cavapoo and they have taken over. They may then loudly verbalize their frustration and displeasure because, in the dog world, the pack follower (which you have allowed yourself to be) does NOT leave the pack leader (them). *I've seen this type of situation many times over, and once the human side of the relationship steps up and takes control, it quickly reverses.*

Breaking your dog of the habit of loud barking when they are left alone can be solved in different ways, with the most obvious being that you simply take your dog with you wherever you go, because after all, they are pack animals, and in order for them to be really happy and well balanced, they need the constant direction of their leader (which is supposed to be you).

Another much more lengthy and time consuming way to solve a barking problem, could involve hiring a professional to help assess why the problem has occurred in the first place and then devise an effective plan to reverse the problem that will work for each unique situation.

Fear or Pain: another reason your dog may bark is when they are very frightened or in pain and this is usually a type of bark that sounds quite different from all the others, often being a combination of a bark and a whine, or a yelping type of noise.

This is a bark that you will want to pay close attention to, so that you can quickly respond and offer the assistance that your puppy or dog may need.

Whatever reason your dog may be barking for, always remember that this is how they communicate and *"tell"* us that they want something or are concerned, afraid, nervous or unhappy about something, and as their guardians, we humans need to pay attention.

Raised Hackles: when your dog approaches with raised hackles (the hair along the dog's back), while this can be an indication that the dog may be approaching with dominant or aggressive tendencies, it also may be an indication that he or she is excited, fearful, startled, anxious or lacks confidence.

In any of these circumstances (whether it's your dog or someone else's), it's a good idea to be respectful and keep your distance until you can assess what's really going on, because even a reactive, fearful dog can quickly turn into a biting dog, and I can tell you from personal experience that being bitten by any dog really hurts.

In a Nutshell

Learning your Cavapoo's particular body language can take some time, and this Chapter will help you get started. The more you are out and about with your dog, visiting and socializing in local parks and going on walks where you will find other dogs, animals and people to observe, the more opportunity you will have to become skilled at recognizing the many subtleties of dog body language.

Paying attention to your Cavapoo's verbal and body-language signals as explained above, will help you figure out what message they are trying to get across to you and this can make all the difference in preventing frustration for you both while raising a happy and well-behaved dog.

One last thought about body language and energy – check in with yourself before you walk out the door with your dog, because if you're not in the moment and have your mind on something that has nothing to do with having a successful and pleasant walk with your dog, you may be setting yourself up for trouble.

For example, if you go out the door with your dog while displaying sad, weak or confusing energy, your dog will pick up on this and become nervous or confused themselves because your energy is no longer conveying to your dog that you are their leader. This means that your energy can literally be the cause of, for instance, an uncomfortable encounter with another person walking their dog.

It's very important to keep in mind that when walking with a dog, the moment they sense that you are not completely in control, they will take this unspoken "cue" from you that being in charge has now defaulted to him or her.

You never want any dog to feel they must protect you from the postman, neighbor's cat or that taunting little Chihuahua in the pink tutu walking across the street, because if they do, you're literally out walking with a highly unpredictable, live "weapon" that could decide to go off at any moment.

Most Cavapoos are pleasant with other dogs and friendly with people, if they have been properly socialized and trained. However, should you permit your dog to get seriously out of control, you could end up with a lawsuit on your hands, and/or sky-high veterinary bills if this little companion is forced into being confrontational with a much bigger dog, and that's if you're lucky.

While this is highly unlikely with a sensitive and friendly Cavapoo, it's still good to keep in mind that if your dog harms another dog, animal or person, the consequences could be far worse than a high vet bill. For instance, any dog that bites could face a death sentence or a ruling that they can never be seen in public unless they're wearing a muzzle.

Chapter 12: Training Basics for a Happy Cavapoo

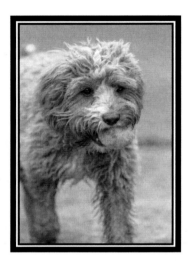

"Everyone thinks they have the best dog in the world. None of them are wrong."
— Unknown

It's no surprise that a properly trained dog will be a much happier, safe and more secure companion that everyone enjoys being around, and that will be far less likely to develop behaviour issues later in life.

When your dog respects your leadership and there is no question that YOU are in charge, your dog can then relax and let you take the lead on training them, which is as it should be. Developing a basic training program and learning to teach your Cavapoo commands and discipline is all part of starting your dog off on the right paw.

Therefore, this Chapter will focus on training basics and tips, including hand signals, as well as simple tricks that your dog will love to learn. Take heed humans, because you will be very happy you spent the time to learn everything contained in these pages.

All of our canine companions are amazing, natural athletes and because of this, no matter their size or breed, they need daily exercise to stay fit and healthy, so that they can be happily well-mannered, and part of their exercise routine includes learning at least three very important training basics, which are **"Come – Sit – Stay"**.

Every dog will require daily exercise to stay happy and healthy. They will love going for hikes, walks and little adventures with you. Your dog may even enjoy learning routines, tricks, and fun canine sports with their guardian as well as playing and socializing in a pack of other smaller dogs.

Any type of disciplined exercise you can engage in with your dog will help to exercise both their body and their mind and will burn off pent-up daily energy reserves, so that your dog will be a happy and contented companion that is relaxed and not suffering health issues from being overweight.

If you find that your dog is being a pest by chewing inappropriate items around the home or being demanding of your time, or especially unruly when visitors come to call, this is likely because their mind is not being challenged enough or their body is not being exercised often enough, or long enough each day to drain out their daily pent-up energy reserves.

A healthy, adult Cavapoo will thrive when being walked several times each day and may also enjoy the challenge of being engaged in other forms of disciplined canine activity, such as Agility or Trick Training.

This affectionate, intelligent and willing to learn designer dog is a breed of small companion canines that enjoys spending all their time with you, and may be able to excel in several canine sports or even as a therapy dog.

Use your imagination and find out what canine sports your dog may enjoy learning. So long as you prove to him or her that you mean what you say through firm, fair direction and consistency, rather than too many treats, they will not feel the need to manipulate or question your authority, and will happily follow your direction.

Even at the young age of eight to ten weeks, most dogs are capable of beginning to learn anything you can teach. If you wait until they are six months old before beginning any serious training program, you could already have a stubborn problem on your hands and a spunky little dog that may be unwilling to heed your commands.

The backbone of helping to develop a well-balanced and happy Cavapoo is to provide them with a routine that ensures sufficient time to satisfy their particular physical and mental exercise needs, in combination with additional time to play, sniff, search and explore their world every day.

What you can teach this canine companion depends entirely upon you and the time and patience you have to devote to their education, and you never want to under estimate what incredible hidden talents your dog may have.

For instance, this outgoing and happy little *hybrid* can be both glamorous AND athletic. Hiding underneath that beautiful, silky coat is a strong and muscular body, and an intelligent mind. For instance, this dog definitely has the potential to be your very own Agility, Trick or Advanced Obedience champion.

No matter what you decide to teach your dog, always train with patience, kindness and positive rewards.

All training sessions should be happy and fun-filled with plenty of food rewards and positive reinforcement, which will ensure that your dog is a happy, attentive student who trusts and respects you as their leader and looks forward to learning new commands, tricks and routines.

Cavapoo Puppy Training Basics

First, choose a *"Discipline Sound"* that will be the same for every human family member. This will make it much easier for your Cavapoo puppy to learn what they can or cannot do and will be very useful when warning or redirecting your puppy before they engage in unwanted behavior.

The best types of sounds are short and sharp, so that you and your family members can quickly say them and so that the sound will immediately get the attention of your puppy, as you want to be able to easily interrupt them when they are about to make a mistake.

It doesn't really matter what the sound is, so long as it gets your dog's attention and everyone in the family is consistent. A sound that is very effective in most cases is a simple *"UH!"* sound that is said sharply and with emphasis.

Most puppies and dogs respond immediately to this sound and if caught in the middle of doing something they are not supposed to be doing, they will quickly stop and give you their attention or back away from what they were doing.

Next, your puppy needs to learn the Three Most Important Words, which are *"Come"*, *"Sit"* and *"Stay"*. These three basic commands will ensure that your puppy remains safe in almost every circumstance.

For instance, when your puppy correctly learns the *"Come"* command, you can always quickly bring them back to your side if you should see danger approaching. Also, when you teach your puppy the *"Sit"* and *"Stay"* commands, you will be further establishing your leadership role, and a puppy that understands that their human guardian is their leader will be a safe and happy follower.

Most puppies are ready to begin training at approximately 10 to 12 weeks of age (and some even earlier), so make your training sessions no more than 5 or 10 minutes (2 or 3 times a day), positive and pleasant with lots of praise and/or treats so that your puppy will be looking forward to their next session.

Come: while most Cavapoo puppies will be capable of learning commands and tricks at quite a young age, the first and most important command you need to teach your puppy is the recall, or *"Come"* command.

Begin the *"Come"* command inside your home. Go into a larger room, such as your living room area. Place your puppy in front of you and attach their leash or a longer line to their Martingale collar, while you back away from them a few feet.

Say the command *"Come"* in an excited, happy voice and hold your arms open wide. If they do not immediately come to you, gently give a tug on the leash, so that they understand that they are supposed to move toward you. When they come to you, happily praise them and give a treat they really enjoy.

Once your puppy can accomplish a *"Come"* command almost every time inside your home, you can then graduate them to a nearby park or quiet outside area where you will repeat the process and where there are many more distractions. In order to keep yourself and your dog safe, he or she needs to always come to you when asked, despite whatever distractions may be nearby.

You may want to purchase an extra-long, lightweight line (25 or 50 feet), so that you are always attached to your puppy and can encourage them in the right direction should they become distracted by noises, scents and other dogs. Try to choose a time of day when there will be fewer distractions while you are training.

Keep in mind that even after teaching your Cavapoo the *"Come"* command, their nose may take precedence over the commands you are teaching when outdoors if an interesting scent distracts them. Always keep this dog on leash when working in an area where they can easily run off in pursuit of an intriguing scent.

Sit: the "Sit" and *"Stay"* commands are both easy commands to teach that will help to keep your puppy safe and out of danger in almost every circumstance. Find a quiet time to teach these commands when your puppy is not overly tired.

Ask your puppy to "Sit" and if they do not yet understand the command, show them what you mean by gently squeezing with your thumb and middle finger the area across the back that joins with their back legs.

Do NOT just push them down into a sit, as this can cause damage to their back or joints. When they sit, give them a treat and praise them.

When you say the word *"Sit"*, at the same time show them the hand signal for this command. While you can use any hand signal, the universal hand signal for *"Sit"* is right arm (palm open facing upward) parallel to the floor, and then raising your arm while bending at the elbow toward your right shoulder. Once your dog is sitting reliably for you, remove the verbal "Sit" and replace it with the hand signal.

Every time you take your dog out for a walk, which is often a cause of excitement, get into the habit of asking them to sit quietly and patiently at every stage of your walk.

For instance, ask your Cavapoo to sit and patiently wait while you put on their leash, while you put on your shoes or jacket, after you approach the door, after you are on the other side of the door, while you lock the door, every time you arrive at a street intersection or crosswalk, every time you stop during your walk to speak to a neighbor, greet a friend or admire the view, etc., and do this all in reverse when heading back home.

When you persist with the *"Sit"* training, it will soon become automatic for your dog to calmly sit every time you stop walking. When you ask your dog to sit for you, they are learning several things all at once; that they must remain calm while paying attention to you, that you are the boss, that they must look to you for direction and that they must respect you as their leader.

Keep in mind that a sitting puppy is much easier to control than one standing at the alert, ready to bolt out the door or jump on someone. As well, because the action of sitting helps to calm the mind of an excited puppy (or dog), teaching your puppy the *"Sit"* command is a very important part of their daily interactions with your family members as well as people you may meet when out on a walk.

When you ask your puppy to *"Sit"* before you interact in any way with them, before you go out, before you feed them, etc., you are helping to quiet their mind, while teaching them to look to you for direction, and at the same time making it more difficult for them to jump, lunge or disappear out a door.

Stay: once your puppy can reliably "Sit", say the word *"Stay"* (with authority in your voice) and hold your outstretched arm, palm open toward their head while backing away a few steps. If they try to follow, calmly say "No" and put them back into "*Sit*". Give a treat and then say again, "*Stay*" with the hand signal and back away a few steps.

Practice these three basic "*Come*", "*Sit*", "*Stay*" commands everywhere you go, and use the "*Sit*" command as much as you can to ensure its success rate.

As your puppy gets older, and their attention span increases, you will be able to train for longer periods of time and introduce more complicated routines.

Hand Signals

It's really important to use the hand signals that go along with the verbal commands during training, so that once your Cavapoo learns both, you can remove the verbal commands in favor of just hand signals.

Hand signal training is by far the most useful and efficient training method for your dog. All too often we inundate our canine companions with a great deal of chatter and noise that they really don't understand, but because they are so willing to be part of our world, they soon learn the meaning of many words.

Contrary to what some people might think, the first language of a Cavapoo (or any dog) is a combination of sensing energy and watching body language, which requires no spoken word or sound.

Therefore, when we humans take the time to teach our dog hand signals for all their basic commands, we are communicating with them at a level they instinctively understand, plus we are helping them to become a focused follower, as they must watch us in order to understand what is required of them.

Simple Tricks

When teaching your dog tricks, in order to give him or her extra incentive, find a treat that they really like and give the treat as a positive reward, which will help solidify a good performance.

Most dogs will be extra attentive during training sessions when they know that they will be rewarded with their favorite treats – especially this dog, who will usually have a healthy appetite.

If your puppy is less than six months old when you begin teaching them tricks, keep your training sessions short (no more than 5 or 10 minutes) and fun. As they become adults, you can extend your sessions, as they will be able to maintain their focus for longer periods of time.

Shake a Paw: who doesn't love a well-trained dog that knows how to shake a paw? This is one of the easiest tricks to teach your dog.

TIP: most dogs are naturally either right or left pawed. If you know which paw your dog favors, ask them to shake this paw. Find a quiet place to practice, without noisy distractions or other pets, and stand or sit in front of your dog. Place them in the sitting position and have a treat in your left hand.

Say the command *"Shake"* while putting your right hand behind their left or right paw and pulling the paw gently toward yourself until you are holding their paw in your hand. Immediately praise them and give them their favorite treat.

Most smart and willing Cavapoos will learn the "Shake" trick quite quickly, and very soon, once you put out your hand, your dog will immediately lift their paw and put it into your hand, without your assistance or any verbal cue.

Practice every day until they are 100% reliable with this trick, and then it will be time to add another trick to their repertoire.

Roll Over: you will find that just as your dog is naturally either right or left pawed, they will also naturally want to roll either to the right or the left side. Take advantage of this by asking your dog to roll to the side they naturally prefer.

Sit with your dog on the floor and put them in a lie down position. Hold a treat in your hand and place it close to their nose without allowing them to grab it. While they are in the lying position, move the treat to the right or left side of their head (the nose will follow the treat), so that they have to roll over to get to it.

You will very quickly see which side they want to naturally roll to, and once you see this, move the treat to this side. When they roll over to this side, immediately give them the treat and praise them.

You can say the verbal cue *"Over"* while you demonstrate the hand signal motion (moving your right hand in a circular motion) or moving the treat from one side of their head to the other with a half circle motion.

Sit Pretty: while this trick is a little more complicated, and most dogs pick up on it very quickly, remember that every dog is different so always exercise patience.

Find a quiet space with few distractions and sit or stand in front of your dog and ask them to *"Sit"*. Have a treat nearby (on a countertop or table) and when they sit, use both of your hands to lift up their front paws into the sitting pretty position, while saying the command *"Sit Pretty"*. Help them balance in this position, while you praise them and give them the treat.

Once your dog can perform the balancing part of the trick quite easily without your help, sit or stand in front of your dog while asking them to *"Sit Pretty"*. Holding the treat above their head at the level of their nose would be when they sit pretty.

If they attempt to stand on their back legs to get the treat, you may be holding the treat too high, which will encourage them to stand on their back legs to reach it. Go back to the first step and put them back into the *"Sit"* position and again lift their paws while their backside remains on the floor.

Sit Pretty hand signal: hold your straight arm, fully extended, over your dog's head with a closed fist.

Make this a fun and entertaining time for both of you and practice a few times every day until they can *"Sit Pretty"* on hand signal command every time you ask.

A smart young puppy should be able to easily learn these basic tricks before they are six months old and when you are patient and make your training sessions short and fun for your dog, they will be eager to learn so much more.

Adult Training

This is a dog that will thrive when being involved in different training routines and/or canine sports, because it means they are getting to spend fun time close to their humans. Therefore, in order to ensure a happy and healthy dog that will not develop behaviour issues out of boredom or laziness, make sure that you get your dog involved in as much activity as possible, such as Advanced Obedience, Trick Training, Agility or perhaps Freestyle Dance.

When your dog is a full-grown adult (approximately two years of age), you will definitely want to begin more complicated or advanced training sessions.

When you have the desire and patience, you may be surprised at how many commands, tricks, routines or canine sports you can teach a happy, willing Cavapoo who trusts and respects their human guardian.

For instance, you may wish to teach your adult dog more advanced tricks, such as opposite sided paw shakes or rollovers, which are more difficult than you might expect and which the intelligent Cavapoo is definitely capable of learning.

If you and your dog are really enjoying learning new tricks or routines together, consider teaching them a series of hand signals, such as "Commando crawl", "Speak" or "Jump through the human hoop", or perhaps get them certified as a therapy dog so they can brighten the days of those who must spend time in hospitals and care facilities.

Teaching your dog tricks and routines builds trust and respect, is fun for both of you, and a healthy way to exercise both your dog's mind and body, which will result in a happy, contented and well-behaved companion.

Over-Exercising

Be especially careful about over-exercising your Cavapoo when it's warm out and when they are really young (as their muscles and bones are not yet fully developed), because like humans, dogs can also collapse from heat stroke.

Playtime

Every dog needs some down time or regular playtime each day, and while every dog will be different with respect to what types of games they may enjoy, most will really love any game involving retrieving a ball or soft toy.

The smart Cavapoo may also be a very excited participant in a fun game of *"Search"*, where you ask your dog to *"Sit/Stay"* while you hide a favorite treat that they then have to use their nose to find.

To begin teaching the "Search" game, first time ask your dog to sit/stay while you slowly back away and place a treat where they can actually still see it. Return to where they are in their sit/stay and say, "OK! Search!" and point to where you just placed the treat. Each time you play this game, you can place the treat farther and farther away and completely out of their sight before you release them to "Search!"

After a disciplined walk with your dog, they will also enjoy being given the opportunity for some off-leash freedom to really stretch out by running free to play and socialize with other similar-sized dogs at the local dog park.

In a Nutshell

Taking the time to teach your dog basic rules and boundaries, plus simple or complex tricks, will keep them both mentally and physically healthy and happy and you will raise a well-behaved dog that is a joy to be around.

The Cavapoo is a very smart, sturdy and willing to please little dog, which means that in order to ensure a healthy, happy and contented dog that is not overweight and will not develop behavior issues out of boredom or neglect, you must take the time to involve them in daily moderate exercise; that can include different activities, such as interesting canine sports where they get to develop their unique skills.

Chapter 13: What If You Slip Up?

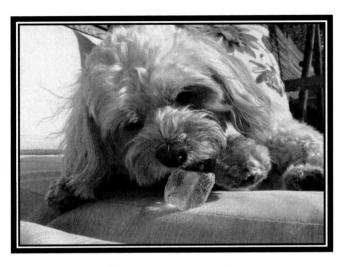

"Dogs got personality.
Personality goes a long way."
— Quentin Tarantino

All the information, suggestions, tips and advice given in this book is the result of more than 40 years experience helping humans positively and effectively interact with the canine world.

If you take all that is written on these pages to heart, and regularly and consistently apply them, your Cavapoo will grow up to be a happy family member that will not have to suffer from any behavioral issues.

However, if your lifestyle drastically changes, you forget to exercise your dog, keep on top of basic or advanced training, or you slip up for any number of reasons, problems may inevitably occur.

For instance, you may end up becoming too busy or distracted with your human life to provide your canine companion with what he or she needs on a daily basis to be a happy and fulfilled member of your family.

Realistically, there may be any number of other reasons why you don't consistently apply the information given here, and the following is an outline of just a few of the more common behavioral issues that may occur, with some tips that may help you get back on track.

When reading the following pages, please keep in mind that a specific behavioral problem is usually the result of many different possibilities or circumstances that have taken place between the human individual or family and the particular dog.

This means that properly addressing a specific unwanted behavior often needs the assistance of a professional with a personal approach, who can ask the right questions to determine how the unwanted behavior occurred, because it's often not what you may have initially thought.

Therefore, to generically outline possible ways to reverse an unwanted behavior will be a guessing game, because without knowing the circumstances of the guardian and their family, and understanding the situation that triggered the unwanted behavior, I can only make my best guess based on previous experience with similar problems.

As an example, there might be many reasons why the Cavapoo in question is chewing the tassels on your Persian rug. For instance, this could be because they:

- are hungry
- are teething
- have a taste for wool
- think the tassels are a toy
- are a super high energy dog
- are left alone and are bored
- haven't been given appropriate toys to chew
- have not been taught rules and what is appropriate
- need a guardian with stronger leadership energy
- are under-exercised
- are over-stimulated

As you can see, it's possible for almost endless scenarios and reasons why a dog may develop a particular behavioral issue.

Therefore, please understand that without close observation and much more information explaining a particular situation, the following few common behavioral problems and the suggestions for alleviating them, will be my best guess.

Chewing Inappropriate Items
[Re-visit *"Distraction and Replacement"* in Chapter 10]

If your puppy or dog is chewing the carpet, your fingers, the legs of the coffee table, or any other inappropriate item(s) that are not dog toys, rather than getting upset with your dog, you need to train yourself to be much more vigilant, and then distract and replace.

First make sure that all the chewing is not just because the puppy is teething. Have compassion because teething is painful for the puppy and they must chew to help alleviate the pain while those adult teeth are growing in.

Always make sure your puppy has plenty of chew toys and to help with the teething pain, give your puppy an old T-towel soaked in water, tied in knots and frozen in the freezer as a chew toy.

When your Cavapoo is a little older, already has pushed through their adult set of teeth and has decided, for instance, that the legs on your coffee table are good chew toys, it is possible that you:

- are not paying attention and taking the time to make sure your dog receives enough daily exercise, and/or,

- are not teaching your dog what is, and what is not, appropriate for chewing by saying a firm and convincing **"No"**, replacing the table leg with a toy they are allowed to chew, and praising them when they've got the right thing between their teeth.

Being Fearful of Loud Noises
[Re-visit *"Fear of Loud Noises"* in Chapter 10]

If you have raised a dog that has a fear of loud, popping noises, perhaps you haven't taken the time to read this information and apply the suggestions outlined, so read it now and practice until your dog loses or at least diminishes their fear.

Excessive Excitement When Friends Visit
[Re-visit *"Chapter 3: Overview of the Happy Cavapoo"* and *"Chapter 12: Training Basics for a Happy Cavapoo"*]

Make sure that you begin to teach an excitable young Cavapoo to be a calm follower as soon as you bring him or her home.

Always ignore an excited dog and do <u>not</u> touch them until they are calm and relaxed, otherwise you will inadvertently teach them that it is acceptable behavior for them to be excited every time they see a human.

If they are overly excited when friends come to visit, stand between your dog and your friends, and create some space by pointing away and firmly telling your dog, *"GO"*, and also ask your friends to ignore him or her.

Also, if you've been properly training your puppy or dog, you will have taught them to *"Sit"* on command, and a sitting dog is much more relaxed and easier to control.

Acting Aggressively on a Walk
[Re-visit *"Chapter 12: Training Basics for a Happy Cavapoo"*]

Make sure that your dog is walking at your side without pulling on the leash when you are out for a walk.

When you train your dog to walk beside you, this "tells" them that YOU are their leader and in charge of every situation, which means they will be much less likely to act out or attempt to "protect" you from outside stimuli. If they DO try, immediately give a sharp snap on that Martingale collar along with a strong *"NO!"* to remind them who is the boss.

Pulling When on Leash
[Re-visit *"The Martingale Collar"* in Chapter 10]

If your dog is pulling on leash, chances are high that he or she is not wearing the proper training collar and you have not taken the time to teach them to quietly walk at your side.

Buy your dog a Martingale collar, properly adjust it, and then the next time they try to pull ahead of you, give a sharp snap to this collar (toward yourself) and firmly say the word "*Heel*".

Repeating this process until your dog understands can take a few minutes or even several days, as each dog is different – be consistent and persistent until your dog gets it.

Also, turning circles and changing directions suddenly when on a leash walk will quickly help to teach your dog their proper walking position, because if they are ahead of you they are going to be stepped on or walked into.

Stealing Food or Raiding the Garbage Can
[Re-visit "*Ideal Living Conditions for a Happy Cavapoo*" in Chapter 6]

Make sure you absolutely understand that while the Cavapoo hybrid may not be a particularly food motivated breed, if given the opportunity and the food is enticing enough, any dog will steal food. This means that in order to avoid this possibility, you must be a vigilant guardian and make sure that you never leave any food they should not eat unattended or where they can reach it.

Not Obeying Commands
[Re-visit "*Chapter 12: Training Basics for a Happy Cavapoo*"]

A well-trained Cavapoo is one that obeys the basic "*Come/Sit/Stay*" commands. If your dog is not obeying your commands, you have not taken the time to properly train them, or you are too weak a leader, with the result being that he or she will take a stubborn attitude, they will ignore you and they will not respect you as their leader. Get to work right away, step up your energy to ensure you are a strong enough leader, and train your dog so that everyone will be happy.

We all have our off days, so don't get down on yourself if you occasionally slip up and are not being as vigilant, strong and confident a leader as you need to be with this dog's basic and/or advanced training and daily maintaining of rules and boundaries.

In a Nutshell

We humans will always have days when we are not as vigilant as we need to be, which means that we will inevitably "slip up" sometimes when raising our fur friends.

What you need to remember is that it's not the end of the world, because there is always a solution, and often simply re-reading the relevant chapters in this book can quickly and easily get you back on track to raising a happy and well-behaved Cavapoo that is a pleasure to be around.

Also, know that the familiar expression *"You can't teach an old dog new tricks"* is totally false. It doesn't matter what age a particular dog may be, because with the right knowledge, you absolutely CAN teach a dog of any age new tricks.

Chapter 14: Surprise Bonus Chapter

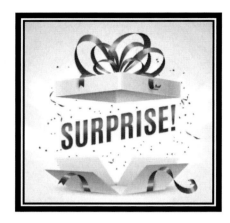

"Dogs have a way of finding the people who need them, and filling an emptiness we didn't ever know we had."
— Thom Jones

If you thought that you had reached the end of this book, well surprise, not quite yet, as I'd like to leave you with some canine wisdom and a short, funny, true story.

Happy Cavapoo Question and Answer (Q&A) section

The following Question and Answer (Q&A) section is written from the dog's perspective, and although you may find it amusing, there are also valuable human lessons to be learned, if anyone is paying attention.

First, let me set the scene for the following situations:

This is a young, busy family, consisting of Mom and Dad, who work at home, one 12-year-old girl, and one 14-year-old boy, who share their lives with a neutered, 2-year-old dog named Harvey. They all live together in a large house with a medium-sized, fenced yard out the back.

The following questions, asked by various members of the family, are directed to the dog, and answered by the dog, as if the dog could talk like their humans.

Each question that the dog answers is followed by a short synopsis of the "lesson" we humans can learn from these various interactions.

Mom: **"Oh No! Why did you pee on the floor?"**

Harvey: *"Ah, maybe because I drank a bowl of water after my dinner, and you forgot to let me out before everyone left for that baseball game, and I just couldn't hold it any longer."*

Lesson: Humans often lead very busy lives, and in order to ensure their dog remains happy, they still need to always pay attention and put their canine friend's habits and needs ahead of their own.

Girl: **"Yuckeeee! Harvey, why do you smell like dog poo?"**

Harvey: *"Could it be because, as much as I tried to tiptoe through those piles of doggy doo in the back yard, that as far as I'm concerned smell much better than tulips, I got distracted by that taunting squirrel and accidentally stepped in one."*

Lesson: Humans with convenient back yard doggy bathrooms often forget to be vigilant about picking up the yard. This is not only a smelly bad habit that busy (or lazy) guardians are guilty of, it's also a considerable health hazard that attracts rats.

Boy: **"What's wrong, Harvey? You like to fetch — go get that ball!"**

Harvey: *"Yes, I like to fetch, but it's hot out here, and I'm getting exhausted."*

Lesson: Sometimes we humans that share our lives with short-nosed dogs that have compromised breathing tend to forget that the temperature of the day that doesn't seem extreme to us, can quickly be too much for a dog that is running back and forth fetching a ball. We also forget that many dogs, despite their discomfort, may continue to fetch that ball even though they may be about to collapse from heat exhaustion.

Dad: **"What happened in here, Harvey! You've made a huge mess of all these boxes I had neatly stacked in the carport! What's wrong with you?"**

Harvey: *"Wait a minute - nothing wrong with me! There was a squirrel in here eating through the boxes and I was just trying to protect the home. I finally got rid of him, and he won't be coming back, so don't blame me for that irritating squirrel's antics. You should be thanking me."*

Lesson: Often we tend to quickly blame our canine friends when a mess is created for which there seems to be no explanation. We need to first think beyond simply blaming the dog for unexplained disarray, as there is often a good explanation that, in most cases, exonerates your canine companion.

Mom: **"Harvey! What have you done? I left a plate of butter on the coffee table. Did you eat it?"**

Harvey: *"Thanks for leaving that out for me. It tasted really good and I sure enjoyed it at the time, but now I'm feeling a little under the weather."*

Lesson: Many of our canine companions don't know when to stop when it comes to filling their stomach. Therefore, if you have one of these dogs with an endless appetite for anything remotely resembling food, you need to be vigilant about never leaving kitchen food, garbage or anything edible where they can reach it.

Boy: **"You bad, bad dog, Harvey! You've ruined my expensive tennis shoes."**

Harvey: *"What's the big stink about? You gave me your old shoes to play with, and now you're mad at me? Someone's confused."*

Lesson: Think about what you allow your canine friend to play with, because giving them old discarded shoes, socks or other articles of clothing, etc., to play with causes confusion in the canine mind when you get mad if they decide to chew your new shoes.

Girl: "You're covering my bed in mud, Harvey! Get out!"

Harvey: *"Forget it! You let me sleep in your bed when I was a puppy, so move over and let me in."*

Lesson: If you'd rather not share your bed with a dog that could have just walked through a big mud puddle, don't make the mistake of allowing them to sleep with you when they're a cute and much smaller cuddly puppy. If you do, it's unfair to blame your canine companion for wanting to continue this habit that you literally taught them.

Dad: "Are you kidding me, Harvey! There were three hot dogs on the picnic table!"

Harvey: *"I saved them from the circling crows and ate them while you were getting a beer. Delicious they were - got any more?"*

Lesson: Dogs are carnivorous and no matter their size, whether a tiny Chihuahua or a large Mastiff, if given the opportunity, their desire to eat meat is a strong instinct they cannot ignore. If you leave meat unattended, and your dog eats it, too bad stupid human - don't blame your canine companion.

Moral of the Q&A section

Always DO pay attention to what your dog is trying to tell you, because (in addition to the above), there are so many other lessons we humans can learn from our beloved canine companions. Watching out and learning these lessons, and appropriately acting upon them, will help you to raise a Happy Cavapoo that will never have to experience unwanted behaviors.

There are so many lessons we humans can learn from our beloved canine companions IF we are paying attention.

Happy Cavapoo True Story

Before we close this Chapter, I hope you will enjoy the following true short story:

Ozzy's New Tiles

I was dog-sitting Ozzy for clients of mine who had just recently installed a new tile entranceway in their home where previously there had been carpet tiles. The owners warned me that they were having a *"little problem"* getting Ozzy used to the new, shiny and quite slippery tiles and I told them not to worry about it, as I presumed this was a minor issue.

However, I soon found out that the joke was on me, because once I had delivered Ozzy's owners to the airport and I returned to the home with Ozzy on leash at my side and I opened the front door, I was brought to a sudden abrupt halt when Ozzy refused to enter the house.

Ozzy stopped so suddenly that all the groceries I was carrying became airborne and ended up strewn across the floor while it felt like I had suddenly become attached to a fire hydrant. OK, so much for the *"little"* problem Ozzy was having with the new flooring because he flatly refused to put even one paw on those shiny new tiles.

Thank goodness it was a pleasant summer day because now was the time to start working out Ozzy's fear of shiny surfaces and this meant keeping the front door open.

I tied Ozzy's leash to the railing near the door, rescued my groceries from the tiled floor, found some of Ozzy's favorite treats, and returned to untie Ozzy while I showed him I had treats. He was immediately interested in the treats and started to follow me into the house only to abruptly stop at the door.

I went inside a couple of feet and sat down with his treats on the tiled surface, holding my hand out to offer him a treat. He stretched as far as he could without stepping on the tiles trying to get to the treats he really wanted, while I kept calmly encouraging him to move forward.

Finally, after several failed attempts to get him to put a paw on the dreaded tile surface, he completely flattened himself onto his belly and used his legs like a frog to *"swim"* his way across the tiles to get the treats I was offering.

This was definitely one of the funniest things I had ever seen a dog do, but I had to be careful not to laugh because he needed me to be his strong and confident leader, so I stifled my laughter and praised him for being so brave.

So now here was Ozzy flat on his belly in the middle of the shiny tile surface with his beloved carpeting about ten slippery tiles away. I stood up and moved farther into the house onto the carpeted area, still encouraging him to come and get his favorite treats.

He looked up at me with those big pleading eyes that seemed to say *"help me out of this predicament"*, and all I could do was talk softly and confidently to him, pretending everything was just fine as I asked him to come and get his treats.

After a couple of minutes, Ozzy decided that the only way to get what he wanted was to *"swim"* a little farther and he flailed with his front paws and kicked with his back feet like a frog until he made his way onto the carpet, where he immediately bounded into life.

Stifling my laughter, I immediately praised and petted him, gave him several of his favorite treats, and all was now right in Ozzy's world, until it came time to go out for a lunchtime walk around the block.

I hitched up Ozzy's leash to his Martingale collar and started to walk toward the front door, which involved crossing over the tiled entranceway, hoping he would forget about his fear, but as soon as we reached the edge of the carpet, he immediately put the brakes on.

I stopped with him, keeping some forward tension on his leash, as I offered him a treat if he would just take one step onto the tiles. Instead, he immediately dropped onto his belly again, like a penguin about to slide down a snow bank, and started pushing himself across the tiles to get to the treat I was offering.

Such a sight he was and so determined to get his treat without having to walk – you had to give him credit for his amazing ingenuity.

When he got to my outstretched hand and gobbled down his treat, I gently picked him up and placed his feet onto the dreaded tiles and again encouraged him to walk toward me. This time, although he remained crouched low, he gingerly attempted his first step, and then another and another until you could actually see a light bulb go off in his little doggy brain when he realized that the smooth surface of the tiles was indeed safe to walk on.

I happily praised him for his bravery and gave him another treat, and then a few more times in and out the door and although he would slightly hesitate when stepping onto the tiles, and stoop down to sniff them, within three days of practicing our little routine, the dreaded slippery tile flooring was no longer a problem for this comical little character.

When his owners returned from their holiday, you can imagine how happy they were to know that they no longer had to carry Ozzy across their entranceway.

Lesson to learn: No matter the age of your dog, and how much you may have socialized them, when you change something in their world, they can become nervous, scared and traumatized. The only way to work through this is with much patience and understanding, coupled with persistent calm energy, and of course, favorite treats.

Chapter 15: Conclusion and Reviews

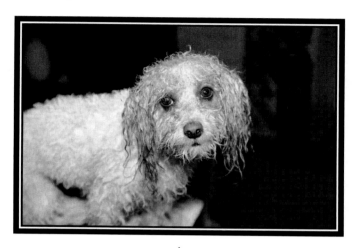

"Once you have a wonderful dog,
a life without one is a life diminished."
— Dean Koontz

This book is written to help anyone thinking of sharing their life with the playful and affectionate Cavapoo, to first understand whether or not they truly have the time, energy and lifestyle that would be compatible with raising a healthy and happy dog.

Once it's been decided that the smart, loving and peaceful Cavapoo is the right breed to share your life with, the purpose of this book is to help you understand how to properly care for them. This will include socializing, training and providing this dog with adequate physical and mental daily exercise, the best food, and a safe environment, so that this dog can live the longest and most contented life possible.

There are already plenty of books written, and many different trainers and opinions concerning how to correct a dog that may be suffering from any number of behavioral issues.

However, to my knowledge, there are no breed-specific books outlining how most, if not all issues are unknowingly created by the dog's human guardian. Therefore, this breed-specific book stands out from all other current publications, because it:

- highlights that almost all problems, both mentally and physically, are a direct result of ignorance or unwillingness on the part of the human guardian to learn what their dog truly needs.

- describes in detail what the human guardian needs to understand and commit to doing on a daily basis in order to match the Cavapoo's needs, so that they can raise a happy, healthy and well-behaved dog that never has to experience behavioral issues.

There is much knowledge for this breed contained within the pages of this book that has been gained over some 40 years working with dogs. This information will help anyone serious about raising a happy Cavapoo, so that they can easily implement all the practical tips of this book without having to hire a professional to help them correct any sort of future behavioral problems.

In a nutshell, this book contains all you need to raise a Happy Cavapoo that will never have to experience unwanted behaviors.

What Past Clients Have to Say

The following are a few happy reviews from some of my past dog whispering clients, who did the work required to turn their Cavapoo into a happy and well-behaved companion. I have taught these clients how to apply some of the tips and techniques described in this book (such as how to establish yourself as the pack leader) and they easily managed to get back on track to raising a happy and well-behaved companion.

Thus, rather than taking my word for the effectiveness of the methods contained in this book, perhaps you would prefer to take my clients' word!!

>*"Thank you for your report and teaching me to be a pack leader ... this has worked remarkably as Drew and Sammy have*

responded well beyond my expectations... Drew is very calm and relaxed and our walks are now very enjoyable...

I want you to know that I really appreciate your help... Results have been spectacular and both dogs have evolved into superheroes and have accepted me as their pack leader and respond positively..."
~ Klaus, Drew, Sammy & Max the Cat

"I just wanted to thank you again for our lesson today. You really are amazing with dogs. Tim and I learned so much from you, it's really neat to see the difference it makes in the dogs when you take control..."
~ Morgan, Tim, Grizzly, Bella & Bear

"I was at the point I was ready to give Jake away because I was so concerned about how he reacted every time someone came to the door. It was really embarrassing! Honestly, within three hours of Asia being here, Jake was a different dog. We learned how to become the pack leader and control him..."
~ Sharon, Mike & Jake

"My partner and I and our dog Rollo recently moved to Victoria from up north. Rollo, unused to city life and walking on a leash, was nervous and reactive around other dogs. Asia showed us how we need to behave so he could relax. After just one session the difference was very impressive – walks have become relaxing and enjoyable again – for all of us..."
~ Tim, Mary & Rollo

"Thank you for helping me become the guardian that Ida needs. She was a good dog to start with, now she is an incredible dog. She walks well on lead, stays in my unfenced yard, and comes when called. I am often complimented on what a well-behaved dog I have. Thanks for making it all happen..."
~ Kristiane & Ida

Published by Worldwide Information Publishing 2020

Made in United States
North Haven, CT
05 June 2022

19873418R00087